REIKI Healing

Learn the Ancient Practice of Reiki Healing to Reduce Depression and Awaken Your Spiritual Energy

(Energy Medicine Guide to Learning Self-healing to Rebalance the Energies)

Steve Keyes

Published by Rob Miles

Steve Keyes

All Rights Reserved

Reiki Healing: Learn the Ancient Practice of Reiki Healing to Reduce Depression and Awaken Your Spiritual Energy (Energy Medicine Guide to Learning Self-healing to Rebalance the Energies)

ISBN 978-1-989990-32-2

All rights reserved. No part of this guide may be reproduced in any form without permission in writing from the publisher except in the case of brief quotations embodied in critical articles or reviews.

Legal & Disclaimer

The information contained in this book is not designed to replace or take the place of any form of medicine or professional medical advice. The information in this book has been provided for educational and entertainment purposes only.

The information contained in this book has been compiled from sources deemed reliable, and it is accurate to the best of the Author's knowledge; however, the Author cannot guarantee its accuracy and validity and cannot be held liable for any errors or omissions. Changes are periodically made to this book. You must consult your doctor or get professional medical advice before using any of the suggested remedies, techniques, or information in this book.

Upon using the information contained in this book, you agree to hold harmless the Author from and against any damages, costs, and expenses, including any legal fees potentially resulting from the application of any of the information provided by this guide. This disclaimer applies to any damages or injury caused by the use and application, whether directly or indirectly, of any advice or information presented, whether for breach of contract, tort, negligence, personal injury, criminal intent, or under any other cause of action.

You agree to accept all risks of using the information presented inside this book. You need to consult a professional medical practitioner in order to ensure you are both able and healthy enough to participate in this program.

Table of Contents

INTRODUCTION 1

CHAPTER 1: BEING ATTUNED TO REIKI 3

CHAPTER 2: HOW TO TREAT YOURSELF WITH REIKI 23

CHAPTER 3: SELF-EXPLORATION 26

CHAPTER 4: THE 3 PILLARS OF MODERN REIKI 45

CHAPTER 5: DE-CALCIFYING THE PINEAL GLAND 61

CHAPTER 6: TYPES OF REIKI HEALING 70

CHAPTER 7: UNDERSTAND THE LEVELS OF REIKI 76

CHAPTER 8: THE POWER OF ATTUNEMENTS 80

CHAPTER 9: HEALING OTHERS & ANIMALS 97

CHAPTER 10: ANGEL JAR 104

CHAPTER 11: BENEFITS FROM INCREASED REIKI EFFORTS 115

CHAPTER 12: REIKI LEVEL 2 119

CHAPTER 13: HEAL CHAKRAS AND REALIGN YOUR ENTIRE CHAKRA SYSTEM 123

CHAPTER 14: REIKI SYMBOLS 135

CHAPTER 15: NUMBER OF REIKI 146

CHAPTER 16: THE POWER OF HEALING 164

CHAPTER 17: SPIRITUAL CONNECTIONS 181

CONCLUSION 192

Introduction

The universe, most especially planet earth is blessed with various gift from God which are most of the time left untapped by human being. We know of Electrical Electronics Energy being used to power electronics, Energy of gravity pulling downward and keeping object stationed to the earth, that of magnetism which is of attraction between two or more objects and radiation which is the transmission and emission of energy in the form of particles or waves through an atmosphere or through any material. From western knowledge, our body house most of these energies which are the significant basis of human physical existence.

Generally, people are looking for ways to get eased-off of stress developed in our body through daily activities. But finding the right medicine to help achieve this has been a tiring task since a very long time. With this book you will be able to help yourself and others who might be in need of stress relief.

Reiki is being defined and re-explained in most chapters of this book, which will allow you understand more, the meaning of Reiki.

I'm positive you will be left astonished learning or using this healing technique

Chapter 1: Being Attuned To Reiki

Up until now, the only way you could have been attuned to Reiki was if you attended classes run by an existing Reiki Master.

Now this was fine, as far as it went. Indeed, we taught Reiki in this way ourselves for many years.

But the problem was this...

It precluded everyone who couldn't afford the very high fees.

And this is very unfortunate. For it's our belief that the world is crying out for the kind of help which people attuned to Reiki can give.

And it's help which needs to be given right NOW.

We cannot wait a moment longer.

The more people able to attune themselves to the energy of Reiki, the better off we all will be.

How so? Well...

There's little doubting that our wonderful planet is presently facing some rather dire problems. And it's no great secret that these problems are beginning to threaten the very survival of humanity itself.

It's also no great secret that it's humanity itself who are creating these problems.

So...

If more people were attuned to Reiki it would begin to raise the consciousness, awareness and understanding of more and more individuals.

And...

As the only way to change the outer world is to first change the inner world of each individual person, it follows that the more internal worlds changed by Reiki the more quickly the outer world will change too.

This is why we decided to share, within the pages of this book, our extremely powerful self-attunement process, so you can attune yourself to the fabulous energy of Reiki right now.

And we make no apologies for doing so.

Yes, we're acutely aware the Reiki purists will throw up their arms in horror.

They'll claim this should never have been done – it's not right – it's not proper etc.

But that's okay; in time they'll come to appreciate the necessity for it.

For the survival of our world needs everyone to have Reiki now, not at some distant time in the future. Reiki is a living, growing, ever expanding art – it cannot be left in the hands of just the few.

Welcome to the Reiki Revolution

This book has been written, therefore, with the intention of changing your life and the direction of our world forever.

We want you to read it and feel...

Wow, I can do this – I have to do this.

Our aim is to inspire you to discover Reiki for yourself and to encourage you to begin walking your own Reiki path.

Notice we say your own Reiki path because Reiki, as far as we are concerned, is all about freedom.

Freedom to become who you want to become and to live your life the way you want to live it.

The way life is supposed to be lived.

In other words Reiki will help guide you towards living the kind of life you may only have dreamed of living.

And this book, we hope, will help guide you towards your own Reiki.

A Word of Warning

However before you go any further we feel compelled to issue you with the following warning…

Please do not expect a solemn, dusty old tome, which tells you exactly how to live your life.

This book will never do that.

You see that would just disempower you - and we have no wish to do this.

We want to fill you with a true sense of your own magnificence and, most importantly, a grand understanding of your own absolute, inviolate, impeccable sovereignty.

Oh yes, one other thing, before we move on.

This book may challenge your present way of thinking, so we would just like you to consider this…

Your mind is like an umbrella in the rain - if it's open it works, if it's closed… well, it just doesn't.

Our intention

Our goal, then, is to provide a solid platform of understanding from which you can go on to build and develop your own dynamic belief system.

And this is a very important point.

For we do not want to enforce our belief systems on anyone.

What works well for us might not necessarily work as well for you.

Truth, as you will discover, is not absolute. What's true for you today might not be true tomorrow.

So, we prefer the idea of providing roots and wings.

Roots to keep you grounded in reality - wings to help you fly through dreaming glorious dreams.

You see, this is one of the major problems with life today. People don't have dreams anymore.

Depression is at epidemic levels because of this.

People either don't have dreams or, if they do, don't believe they can come true.

But people have to have dreams — it's imperative.

And Reiki can help you both create and achieve them.

Now, just a quick word on...

Gurus or Master's

We are most certainly not about becoming your Guru or your Master and taking away your power.

You are your own master and we seek only to help empower you to the point where you understand this quite clearly yourself.

We do not hold with all these different 'societies' and 'associations' that are constantly springing up to encircle and restrict not only the development of Reiki but the development of you as a person as well.

It is not our intention to form any sort of elitist 'club' of which membership is compulsory.

Independence

Independence, on the other hand, certainly is what we are about.

We are of the opinion that powerful, knowledgeable, independent Reiki Masters are a must and a veritable boon to the world and, indeed, the planet itself.

A true Guru, Master or leader is merely a signpost pointing the way.

They'll encourage you to look in the direction they're pointing, not to look at their finger.

In other words listen to what they have to say, and if it sounds and feels right, and works for you, then assimilate what they're saying into your life.

They're not looking for followers, they're not asking you to just sit at their feet revering them, thinking how wonderful they are.

These people know you can be, and want you to become, the same as they are.

They seek only to empower you.

We don't want you to become a follower of anyone or, indeed, anything.

For YOU are the power.

Our aim is to encourage and empower you towards that realisation.

Some people give away their power to a technique or a ritual. They think it's the technique, ceremony or ritual etc which gives them the power or ability to do whatever it is they're wanting to do.

This is a total misunderstanding and we want you to see through it right away.

Take, for example, the process of…

…Candle magic

In candle magic you're told to buy candles of a certain color for the various different ceremonies you wish to perform. Red for achieving one type of magic spell, green for another, black for something else etc.

You have to prepare an altar in a part of your house and treat the area with great reverence.

The particular ceremony you wish to carry out, for whatever it is you wish to achieve, has to be performed on a certain day or night at a certain time.

You have to cleanse your body in a certain way and dress in a certain colour and sometimes at particular times, you may even have to be naked.

The particular candle or candles, which you are going to use, have to be cleansed and purified in a certain way and are then written on with a needle or similar device.

You write on them whatever it is you wish to achieve, usually three times, and then...

You place these candles on your altar.

At the appropriate time you have to go to your altar and taking your candle or candles, whatever is appropriate, you intone the particular incantation, place the candle in the correct position on the altar and light it.

All of the above is carried out in secrecy and total reverence...

And, if the ceremony has been performed correctly, you are told, you will be successful.

Doesn't that sound great? It might even be worth having a go ourselves, eh!

What do you think?

No, we're only joking; don't go out buying any candles.

Just be aware that these ceremonies can and very often do accomplish what they set out to accomplish.

But, the important thing is to understand how and why they work.

It's not the ceremony that makes the spell work - it's YOU.

It's all about you

Everything about the ritual is designed to focus you on what you want to accomplish.

All the various tasks you have to perform work to affirm, and reaffirm, your singular intention.

They engender within you a deep belief in the outcome.

You intend, and believe, the spell will work - and so it does.

But it's purely your intention and belief.

YOU are the magic.

The ritual and ceremony itself is really just the window dressing, it helps to generate the belief, but...

It's not the important thing.

It's not important, either, which colour candles you have or whether you have any candles at all. It doesn't really matter what time of the day, day of the month, what you are wearing or even whether you are using an altar.

All of these things are quite unimportant in themselves. All of these things can be taken out of the equation and the spell will still work.

The only thing that cannot be taken out of the equation is YOU.

It's YOU, your belief and your intention – they're the important things.

The Message

So, are you getting the message loud and clear?

YOU are the power in your life. YOU - just - YOU.

There is nothing and no-one more powerful than you.

Okay, now before we move on to the Reiki itself, which we will do soon enough - honest, we think it would be advantageous to have a little delve beneath the surface of some…

More esoteric matters

So how about starting the ball rolling with a nice, easy to get your head around subject like…

Where do we come from and why are we here???

Could be good for a few sentences don't you think?

Long, long ago in a time before time, there existed an extraordinarily powerful energy source which began speculating about who and what it was.

It began to wonder about...

Okay, okay... we'll leave it there – sounds too much like the beginning of a science fiction novel doesn't it?

But is it too far from the truth? Let's try this...

In the beginning

If you were to try imagining back to what it must have been like in the beginning.

Right back to the very, very beginning of time, yes even before television.

What would you come up with?

What do you think, what do you feel, would have been taking place?

Just for the next couple of minutes, close your eyes and give it a try.

What, back so soon? Have you given it a go?

Come on now, you can be honest with us. Did you, really? Or are you just happy to read on and let us give you some of our thoughts on the matter?

It's quite okay. We realise that some of you will have given it a quick go, but probably most of you didn't.

And that's fine. It's just the way it should be.

Drifting back in time

Okay, so let's go together. Let's get ourselves comfortable, and drift slowly back in time using our imaginations.

Back, back, slowly back.

Let all of recorded history, the personal history you remember and the cosmic history you don't, just rewind in your head.

Where do you imagine we would be?

What can you see?

Are we still standing on a planet? If so, we haven't gone back far enough yet.

We've got to go back before the existence of matter.

We've got to go way, way back to before the universe began.

Now, what do you imagine there would be, back before the universe began?

Are we still in our bodies? Got to go back further.

Is there still a we? Got to go back even further.

Now, is there just a you? Are you still in a body? If so, go back a tiny bit more.

Is there just the purity of you there now? Just your consciousness, your energy? Are you still there?

Is there anything else?

Okay hold on to this thought, this feeling, for a moment.

If you've really got into this last piece of dialogue, and we mean really got into it, you might have noticed something or felt something, quite profound.

If you have, excellent, if not just bear with us a little bit longer whilst we tell you a story that might just help.

A personal story

And this story just happens to be about me, Chris, one of the writers of this book.

When I was growing up my family weren't particularly religious in any noticeable way. We didn't go to church or Sunday school and I don't remember seeing any religious icons in the house.

However, when I was about nine or ten, I asked my mother what would happen to me when I died.

Her reply shocked me to my core.

She said, "There won't be a you any more, when you're dead, you're dead".

I thought she was just joking with me, and waited for her to laugh, but she didn't. She was quite serious. This was her belief, and she had no trouble in passing it on to me.

For me it was one of those moments, you know the type I mean; one of those real key moments in life that rocks your very foundations.

To my mother it was nothing; she just whisked away and got on with her day.

But I was left devastated.

The statement gnawed at me all through the rest of the day, and going to bed that night was, well... a nightmare.

I didn't dare go to sleep in case I died, and there would be nothing else.

It was dreadful, and I didn't know what to do.

Trying to imagine being dead

This went on for weeks and weeks.

At night I'd lie in bed for ages trying to keep myself awake...

Because, for some reason, I only seemed to think I'd die if I went to sleep.

Every night I'd lie there trying to imagine what it would be like to be dead.

Trying to imagine what it'd be like if there was no more me.

No more me!

Nothing!

Nothing at all, but blackness - for all eternity!

It must have begun to take its toll on me physically, but no one appeared to notice.

I don't remember anyone taking me to one side and asking me if everything was all right, and I didn't dare discuss it with anyone else in the family.

My mother was always right.

Everything changed

Then, one night, whilst I was going through the awful imaginings of total blackness and total nothingness for ever and ever, a little light of understanding came on in my head.

Perhaps it was a satori, a fleeting moment of enlightened thought, because nothing ever seemed so dark and black afterwards.

For I suddenly realised that in all the nights of horror I'd gone through, trying to imagine total nothingness - there was always a part of me observing it all.

A part of me that could not be extinguished no matter how hard I tried!

I suddenly knew, with absolute certainty that a part of me would not, indeed could not, ever die!

It was a moment of total exhilaration.

All the dark horrors were forced away. There now seemed to be a light shining within my head, and it was wonderful.

I could never, ever die. I was immortal - the realisation was almost overwhelming.

I wanted to shout it out loud, to tell everyone, but I couldn't. The sad fact was I didn't have anyone to share it with; I had no one who I could tell.

In fact I've only ever shared this with just a tiny handful of people, and now I've shared it with you.

Back to the script

So, back to that thought we were holding from several paragraphs ago. The profound thought or feeling you may have had is the very same one I had all those years before.

There's a part of you that cannot be extinguished, a part of you that is always observing, a part of you that's always there, a part of you that never dies.

You can travel right back in time in your imagination, as we have just done, or you can do it the scary way I did it as a child, by trying to imagine yourself dead.

It doesn't really matter which way you try...
What you'll find is the same. You cannot disassociate yourself from existence.
You cannot - not be!

Chapter 2: How To Treat Yourself With Reiki

Reiki begins with self-treatment, and unless you yourself are whole and healthy, it is difficult to help others become likewise whole and healthy. Reiki practitioners are advised to treat themselves everyday first thing in the morning, preferably on an empty stomach—so it's best to do it before breakfast.

While the attunement process is considered an important first step, there are some who believe it can be dispensed with unless you seek to help others, as well. For just yourself, however, the following ritual is believed to confer many physical, mental, psychological, and spiritual benefits.

Please note that the word "ritual" here has no religious connotations, whatsoever. It is used in the same way that one would use the word "habit." When you know the steps to something by heart (such as driving, bicycling, or even brushing your teeth), you no longer need to deal with uncertainty. Mastery of the steps allows you to stay focused on the end result and not on the process.

Since reiki works on the understanding that health and well-being are our default states, understanding how the process works is simply not necessary. There's a higher power which seeks to keep us in balance and running at optimal energy levels. One must simply trust in that power and in one's inherent ability to tap into that power.

Some prefer to do the session lying down, some just before they get up out of bed or even open their eyes. Others prefer to sit on a chair or stool. Since your legs should never be crossed, sitting on the floor in lotus posture is not recommended.

The important thing is to make the practice work for you by adapting it to your needs, abilities, and circumstances.

Once you come up with a system that works for you, it's best to stick to it like a ritual. Which isn't to say that you can't make changes as the situation demands.

The Reiki Ideals

Many prefer to start a session (either for themselves or for others) by reciting the five ethics Usui recommended. You can either recite the following quietly in your mind or aloud; whichever you're most comfortable with.

"Just for today, I will not be angry. I will not worry. I will be filled with gratitude. I will devote myself to my work and be kind to others"

A variation goes as follows:

"Just for today, I will not be angry. Just for today, I will not worry. I will honor my parents, teachers, and elders. I will earn my living honestly. I will show gratitude to every living thing."

And do try to mean it, since your thoughts and attitude will affect the flow of ki.

Chapter 3: Self-Exploration

You need to make good use of yourself as an individual, and this means you have to know exactly who you are. You must have every single idea about your personality, your mental state, your emotional state, your feelings, and thoughts towards every single situation, your likes, and dislikes, and the kind of people you want to spend your life with. This allows you to take full control of yourself and explore your inner world without facing any difficulties or challenges.

Before you get to explore our inner world, your first have to accept yourself for who you are and feel happy about being you. You can then take full charge or advantage of who you are and use it to achieve your desired goals. Assume you are not you, and this is another person that you have a full idea of everything they are. Use this now to manipulate this person and influence them to like everything you want and do according to your own interests.

By putting yourself in the image of another person and taking advantage of this personality, you find yourself in a position to fully manipulate this character (yourself in this case) and convince them to believe in what you are doing and support you to reach the destination of your target. Take full control of yourself and allow yourself to serve all your interests without going against your instincts. Do what your emotions what you to do, and not what others want you to do.

Self-exploration is the healthiest thing you can ever do to yourself. You will be serving your interests without interference because there's always no second thought involved. There's nothing to stop you from doing what you want to do with yourself because this is "you" you are using to get what you want.

Below are the steps that should be closely followed to effective self-exploration;

Getting to Know You

Picture yourself and learn who you are. Get to know what makes you happy and what spoils your moods. Allow yourself to follow what your mind wants. This will help you realize its impact on your life, and you will be able to tell if this is exactly what you want for yourself or it is the opposite. If this is what you desire then keep it. If it is different from what you want, ignore it and look for what you consider best for you.

Get to know the people you interact with, and those that you want to keep within your circle, as well as the characters that you feel, should be locked out of your circle. Do not accommodate anything that your mind sees as a hindrance to your progress. Maintain only things that contribute to your own progress and keep you moving forward with a lot of ease.

As a person, you should learn to know what you can do without and what you can never do without. Your personal interests, likes, and dislikes should be playing at your fingertips, and your heart should be in a position to only take in what is best for you and lockout anything that is unhealthy for you. By this, moving on with only you're at your top priority and serving all your interests become the easiest task of your life.

When you know yourself well, you will realize that you get too much obsessed with your personality and that you will stop comparing yourself with other people and this is normally because you get to learn your self-worth and understand what you are capable of and the far you can go to achieve what you want.

The Independent Interview

The independent interview is between you and yourself. There are several questions you need to ask yourself like;

· Where do I want to be in life

· What do I need to get to where I want to be

· Can I achieve this alone

· Can I reach my destination without looking up to someone

· What are the challenges involved in the journey of trying to be who you want

· Am I confident enough to face all these challenges

· Am I safe doing what I personally have decided

You then need to answer all these questions honestly without lying because there's no one you are telling but your own self. Faking an answer to these questions is like trying to be fake. You want to fake your personality and your capability.

For you to perfectly move on and record good progress of your plans, you need to be true to yourself during the self-interview. You need to make sure that you do not depend on anyone and that you can achieve everything when you stand alone to face your life. You need to convince yourself that nothing is impossible for you and that you only need yourself in the race of becoming who you desire to be.

The person you admire should be you on a higher level than your current level of life. If you interview yourself and find it true that you can depend only on yourself to achieve what you want and that you surely need no one but you, then you are good to fly to a high level, and nothing can stop you unless you want to stop yourself from doing better.

Passing the independent interview is the first successful step to achieve your dreams. Believe in yourself and aim higher and work towards achieving what you are aiming at. This will change you from being an ordinary person to become the extraordinary person you have always admired and dreamt of being at some point in your life.

The Story of My Life

Your life history is a key element that you can use to explore yourself. Understanding the story of your life, what you passed through that made you who you are, where you began and where you are currently will make you think of nothing else other than making good use of yourself, your time and your strength.

People have different life stories. My story can never be your story, and each of us understands our stories better than the other person does. What you passed through in life should dictate what you do with your life and where you are heading to. You should always aim higher where you were in the past.

When you have a sad life story, then work towards becoming a better person. A happier person that many people could not think you would become. For example, your childhood might be full of suffering. Maybe your parents died, leaving you an orphan with no siblings to look up to. You grew up in the hands of other people who didn't give you the best treatment that you deserve. Maybe these people treated you like a disgrace to them, and you grew up knowing no peace. Now you have to stand again and face all the odds to offer yourself the kind of life you deserve but didn't get the opportunity to live because of the hands that brought you up.

The story of your life should be left fresh and untouched, and every time you think about trying something new, you should aim at changing your lifestyle and not going back to the same kind of struggle that you went through as a little poor helpless child. Changing your lifestyle should be your top priority because you now have full control of yourself and all the decisions that are made concerning you as an individual.

Your life story should not just be a story that is always there to be narrated to every person but should be your self-motivator to help you chase your goals without facing back. You should use your life story to set your targets right and aim at a higher level.

My Target Statement

The target statement, in this case, contains things that you want to achieve with yourself. Your target statement is set by none other than you. You set these statements based on who you were, who you are, and who you want to become. The person you are today is influenced by who you were yesterday, the kind of situations that you passed through and who you will become tomorrow is determined by who you were yesterday, who you are today and what you do today to make your life different from the one that you lived yesterday.

Put yourself in order and flashback to where you came from. Think about the situations back them that resulted in the current state if the life you are in today. Putting this together will help you identify what you have been missing that you surely deserve and will motivate you to explore your capabilities to build the kind of life you want for your future self.

When setting your target statement, you should consider your past experience and your present situation. This statement should include all the rights you deserve that you have never experienced. For example, if as a child you didn't have the opportunity to put on shoes like other children did while you were going to that primary school in your village, and currently at your 20s you miss the opportunity to enjoy life and have fun as your age mates do, then your target statement should include your children living a better life than you did and getting everything they deserve at the right age. It should also include you becoming a better person than you have always dreamt of.

Cultural Exploration

Cultural exploration needs clear knowledge about your cultural background. You first need to understand where you come from and the cultural beliefs of your people. Your cultural beliefs can help you escape some situations that would have had a negative impact on your life. If your cultural beliefs do not allow you to engage in some activities, then the dangers associated with those activities will always be avoided.

As an individual, you should learn and have full knowledge of your cultural background. This will help you in the smooth progress of your activities because you will never have any fear of committing a taboo or even going against your culture in any way. For example, when your culture dictates that you can never get married to someone from a different tribe when you clearly understand and obey your culture, you won't get yourself into trouble with your ancestors by marrying someone of a different tribe without the knowledge if what your culture believes.

You can explore the beliefs of your culture by using them to get yourself what you want or to stop other people from involving you in some situations that you don't want to get yourself involved in.

Cultural beliefs will always protect you, and if you are sharp enough, you can use this to dodge so many events that you don't feel comfortable with.

Inner Conflict

In the process of self-exploration, you must always come head-on with inner conflict. This is normal and should not raise any alarm. Inner conflict always rises from trying to fight your own emotion to lead them in the direction that you want and that you feel will do you better than when you take a different direction. You will have to convince yourself to go towards one direction to be able to achieve what you feel is best for you and have an excess urge to achieve.

Controlling your emotions sometimes becomes hard when you are not in the right state of mind to prevent your emotions from taking over your decisions. Changing your thoughts to focus them all in a single idea must be challenging. However, you will have to bear the challenges involved in order to succeed in your mission of becoming the person you desire to be.

Your inner self will be pushing you towards something that you want so badly, but your other thoughts must always try to differ with your inner self and tell you to take a different direction. The debate within your own thoughts is what will cause conflict in your mind, and you will always remain the judge that makes the final decision of what you are going to do with your life and what impacts does your decision bring to your progress.

Inner conflict can prevent you from achieving what you had planned for when you are not emotionally stable. The constant struggle of your emotions to overpower each other might be difficult for you to handle, and this is what will lead you to an imbalanced state of mind. It can affect your decisions when you don't train yourself to focus on what you want regardless of the situations that chip in.

Look into the Inner Conflicts

For you to move on and explore your inner world, you must closely look into the inner conflicts within you. You need to learn and understand what causes this conflict from within and how you can manage the conflict. Looking into the conflict will help you understand the route from which it is arising. This will help you gather ideas on how you can stop having struggling against your own mind and calming the conflicts that arise from within.

Understanding the inner conflict with you will help you in coming up with possible solutions on how to handle your emotions and thoughts to prevent them from contradicting with one another, leaving you in the middle of mixed feelings and undecided of what next is best for you. Inner conflict, when not well handled, can make someone go insane when the thoughts become too many that they can't handle themselves and have to look for a psychologist to help them come out of the prison of their own minds.

Weak people easily become slaves to the inner conflict within them that they end up having mixed feelings and want to serve all of them at the same time. They are left torn between decisions because these feelings both result from their own thoughts and the urge to want to prosper and take care of the world.

When we closely and keenly look into the inner conflict, we can easily come up with a solution that doesn't hurt our feelings, and that helps us out of a situation smoothly. It will help us to avoid unnecessary thoughts that can result in the failure of our desired goals.

Creative Exploration

Creative exploration is the base of all kinds of exploring anything you want. When you explore any world creatively, we will end up getting what we want with minimum struggle. This normally comes after we have set everything in place, and there's no hindrance left in our way to success. At this level, there's usually no obstacle left to prevent us from getting what we want.

First, we started by getting to know yourself. You get to learn your interests and get familiar with your thoughts, feelings, emotions, and judgment towards different situations. This is what makes it easier for us to understand what we need and use our own minds and feelings to achieve it. It also helps us to get familiar with our personalities that we won't have a difficult time trying to cope up with different situations.

Secondly, we had to conduct an independent interview to assure ourselves that we are independent and that nothing can stand between us and our thoughts to prevent us from getting what we want out of ourselves and not out of them. We have full control of the decisions that we make, and we don't have to consult anyone to approve our minds.

Then there is the part of 'Story of my life' that keeps us motivated towards achieving something that he had long lusted for. The sad story of your past is what makes you aim higher, trying to avoid being in the same situation that made you feel so much unsatisfied. It makes you want to leave a better life tomorrow than yesterday and today.

The story of a person's life helps them in setting a target statement that will ensure that what they end up in is far much different from how they began. It focused on making our dreams come true and make us lead a different kind of lifestyle from what we had experienced earlier. It trains our mind to look through the future and settle in something that is highly benefiting us.

All these aspects of self-exploration lead us to one direction and make us want to always try something new. This is what leads us to creatively explore everything that comes our way. We always want to make good use of all situations and will always find a way of making something beneficial out of every event. We always attempt to see an opportunity out of every situation and always think of utilizing the opportunity to achieve something better out of it

To creatively explore everything, it is advisable to come up with a unique idea out of all situations that, when put together, can yield something productive. Every single idea should be grown to something big and unique that, when well managed, opens a way for a huge opportunity of making life a better thing than ever before. It should always come out with the best feeling at the thought of utilizing an opportunity that was never noticed before and could have been a waste if it was never noticed.

Creative exploration usually come out of big minds that are ever ready to prosper through every little opportunity that comes their way. The big minds will always create great ways out of small ideas that they construct powerfully to show extraordinary creativity. Big minds are said to have big ideas that, when brought together, leads to a fruitful investment of a simple event that no one could ever see or think of as an opportunity to prosper. It is the extraordinary minds that open big gates from an ordinary situation.

Chapter 4: The 3 Pillars Of Modern Reiki

Foundations. Without strong foundations, any structure is doomed to a fate of failure, and a fate where collapsing is not only a possibility but an inevitability. Whether it happens sooner or later, without strong foundations there is no entity that has even a chance of tasting longevity, let alone dream of actually thriving.

There are many energy healing systems in the world right now, some good, some not so much. These systems are determined 'good' or 'bad' not by the modalities that they champion, but by the fruits that they bear. What I mean by this statement, to put it in the simplest of terms, is that effectiveness is king. When it comes to assessing the effectiveness of any energy healing system, we need only to look at the structure upon which they are formed. Some energy healing systems are built upon the precepts of science, and science alone. These systems stem from the seeds of early modern medicine, seeds that were planted hundreds of years ago, and extend right through to what we now call in the US — and most of the civilized world — our healthcare system.

These science-based healthcare systems are truly amazing. By means of harnessing humanity's thirst for knowledge, we as a species have made great strides in both medical understanding and application. We have created numerous medical protocols and treatments to heal many illnesses and diseases, even eradicating some ailments through inoculations and/or precautionary measures. And technologically, we have created and continue to create surgical procedures that result in positive outcomes for the patient, allowing doctors to heal more effectively than ever before.

However, despite the fact that our science-based systems have made leaps and bounds in advancement, they have limitations. You see, our science-based systems focus primarily on the short-term alleviation of suffering within a patient, and they do so while almost ignoring the actual cause(s) of the ailment. In addition, modern medicine aims to provide immediate relief from a medical issue, but doesn't always create a long-term strategy to both prevent a recurrence of the problem and provide a cure. In fact, the term 'cure' is being used less and less by doctors these days. On the surface, it appears they are refraining from the use of the word 'cure' because they do not believe that cures exist. But if we look closer into the subject we find that doctors are refraining from the word "cure" because they are unsure how to bring them about. And the reason for this phenomenon, where modern healers (doctors) are losing touch with finding cures for their patients, is as simple as it is elusive, because their primary focus is fixed upon the effect (illness) and not the cause (factors that instigated the onset of the illness).

In contrast to science-based systems, there are numerous faith-based systems. In these practices, patients are reconnected with the mind/body relationship. These systems educate patients of the fact that any physical ailment they currently have, is almost always a direct result of what they have thought, or have been thinking, consistently. Faith-based healing systems can include mainstream religions like Christianity, Judaism, Hinduism, etc. They can also include healing arts such as yoga, pilates, acupressure, and even self-help books that focus us on taking control of our thoughts and emotions.

These types of faith-based systems do wonders for people. They can allow us to find the answers of why we have certain health issues, and can free us from conditions that have been haunting us for years. They pull us away from the short-term view of our current pain that we seek relief from and allow us to dig deep, allowing us to look for the things we have been doing wrong in our lives that have led us to this point — whether physical or mental. Unlike modern medicine, faith-based systems take a more rounded approach, helping us to draw parallels between how we have been living, and how that has contributed to where we are now.

However, the real problem found within these faith-based systems is that they tend to focus on things in a manner that is almost always completely divorced of science.

For example: if we look at how religions view healing, they put emphasis outside of ourselves, on a higher power or being. This type of thinking, although founded in some truth, is ultimately dangerous. It is so because when we put too much emphasis outside of ourselves, we start to believe that life is out of our control and happening to us — we become victims of randomness. Is there a power outside of us, a power that we can and should call upon? Of course. But this power is not something that parades over us in majesty. In fact, the power we seek is not just outside of us, it is part of us. I will return to this topic very shortly, but before I do, we must analyze another facet of faith-based healing systems; the systems of movement or faith that are not religious, e.g. yoga, pilates, and similar arts.

These healing arts tend to, again, reconnect us with our responsibility of words, thinking, and the effect it has upon our bodies. They, unlike religions, put less emphasis on outer forces of healing and help you look inward for power. However, much like religious-based systems, these faith-based healing systems divorce themselves from the scientific principles upon which modern medicine relies on. This imbalance results in us overreaching, and when we do that, we always risk falling.

At this point, it may appear as if I'm writing off any and every healing-based system, whether scientific or esoteric. But in truth what I'm actually doing is calling you to entertain the need of our minds and bodies for balance.

As I mentioned earlier, when we reach out to higher forces in religion, we start to supplicate ourselves. This is bad because when we supplicate, we pay a heavy price. Supplication comes at the price of responsibility, and when we give away our responsibility, then we lose our personal power too.

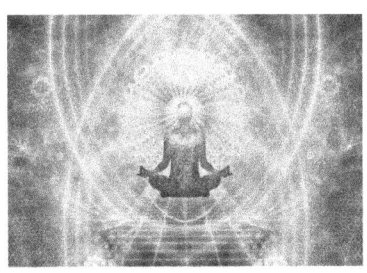

Scientific systems may well have a short-sighted approach to things, but they reconnect us with our human need for exploration and discovery. In essence, they plug us right into the outlet of our own personal power — objective research.

And in contradistinction to the science-based healing systems, faith-based healing systems surrender our responsibility, but also reconnect us with the big picture of everything we say, do, or think, ultimately shaping our emotional and physical wellbeing.

The key, the point of perfect equilibrium, is when science can meet faith, and the two approaches can be melded into a harmonious system.

And this is where Reiki comes into play. Dr. Mikao Usui's Reiki is a system that is based on both science and faith. The system is built upon tenants that encompass both sides of the proverbial coin. Therefore, Reiki has been built on extremely strong, and perfectly balanced foundations, which makes the system applicable and effective for both healers and recipients alike.

Reiki is built upon three pillars: Gassho, Reiji-Ho, and Chiryo.

Let us examine them further.

Gassho

Gassho literally means "two arms folded together". Dr. Usui taught this meditation regularly. It was generally practiced before a Reiki seminar.

As a rule, this type of medication should be practiced for 20-30 minutes after waking up and/or in the evening, before going to bed.

With the help of Gassho meditation, we bring ourselves into a meditative state, a state of unity with the Universe. By joining hands in front of the chest, we help the heart to also tune into the treatment.

Gassho meditation is performed with joined hands in front of your heart with gratitude to God or the Universe.

The attention of the meditator is concentrated to the point of contact between the two middle fingers. In this case, the emerging thoughts float in consciousness, like clouds in a blue sky. We notice them, recognize them, and again shift our attention to the point of contact of the two middle fingers.

In esoteric Buddhism, the left hand represents the moon, and the right hand represents the sun.

Each finger represents one of the Five Elements:
- The thumb represents the Spirit
- The index finger, the Air
- The middle finger, Fire
- The ring finger, Water
- The pinky, Earth

The fingertips represent certain qualities:
- The tip of the thumb represents insight
- The tip of the index finger, the ability to act
- Tip of the middle finger, sensations
- Tip of the ring finger, perception

- The tip of the pinky is the shape

From the point of view regarding the science of meditation, when we put our hands together, we put together the Sun, the Moon, and all the Elements. The circle closes. Focusing on the middle fingers emphasizes the fiery aspect of meditation. Awareness burns the elements of the subconscious.

The fingertips are also the place where many nerves and meridians (energy channels) end. The meridian ending in the middle finger is the meridian of the pericardium in the hand. It passes from the chest along the inner surface of the hand, through the wrist, palm, and ends at the tip of the middle finger.

Most practitioners agree that Gassho's meditation makes it easier to observe our inner dialogue, helping to pause it.

Experience has shown that Gassho meditation is suitable for both the eastern and western mindset, regardless of age, gender, or preparation of the meditator.

Reiji-Ho

Translated into English, **Reiji** means "a sign of Reiki strength," **Ho** means "method".

In the Japanese Reiki tradition, the focus is on the intuitive definition of disharmonious, painful areas on the patient's body (or aura). When we stop the flow of thoughts, the internal speech monologue, and go deep inside ourselves, we can feel what area of the body our hands will "call". It is also the trust of Reiki energy. In the end, it is not ourselves who are treating. The energy is transmitted through us.

Reiji-Ho teaches us to follow our intuition. To follow, not to develop it, because intuition as a divine gift is given to us at birth. Our task is only to learn to hear its voice and do what it tells us.

As for the Reiji technique, just let the energy live freely. Feel like an empty vessel, which itself, without any effort from you, will be filled with vital energy. Do not think about where, when, and how it enters you, everything will happen on its own.

Sit or stand in front of the person you want to heal from some kind of ailment. Close your eyes and fold your hands in Gassho.

Focus your attention in tandem. Let go of any stress and relax. Feel how your body is filled with Reiki energy, and how you become part of this energy.

Ask your patient to be aware of the causes of his ailments and failures. Then ask for his healing at all levels. Slowly move your hands to the "third eye" area and ask Reiki to bring your hands where you need to. Problem areas will call your hands for help themselves.

Now you just have to wait a bit. You will certainly feel where your hands should go. This can happen in different ways. If visual images are closer to you, then you will see the part of the body that needs to be treated. If you tend to perceive the world by ear, you will hear this information. If you are a kinesthetic, that is, you perceive the world as if it were pores of the skin, then you can just feel where you should touch the patient.

You can receive a "message" immediately or after some time. In order to speed up this process, place one or both of your hands on the patient's crown chakra and tune in to the energy of his body.

Regular training will do the trick: you will learn to identify problem areas much faster, and when practicing Reiki for several years, you will see them with a bare glance at the person. You might feel it as a slight tingling sensation in your hands, a feeling of warmth or magnetism, or maybe you will simply realize that the answer is received.

The art of Reiji-Ho is akin to creativity: starting to use it for healing, you can extend your skill to other areas of your life.

Chiryo

Chiryo in English translation means "treatment". At the time of Dr. Usui, treatment was, of course, carried out in a traditional Japanese way.

The patient lay on the floor either on a futon (cotton mattress) or on a tatami (straw bedding). The healer knelt down next to the patient, holding his dominant hand over the patient's parietal chakra until an impulse or inspiration appeared, which the hand would follow.

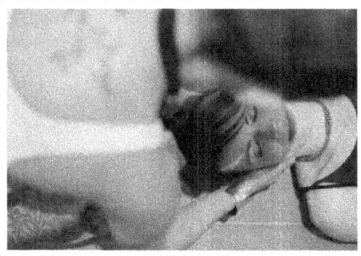

During treatment, the healer gave his hands complete freedom, touching the painful areas of the body until they ceased to hurt or until the hands themselves would move to a new area for treatment.

We will expand on Chiryo later in this book because it is truly the instrument by which

Reiki power is utilized effectively by a Reiki practitioner.

Chapter 5: De-Calcifying The Pineal Gland

The Pineal Gland is not, as we've seen, some esoteric, hard to define, otherworldly concept. It's real, it's pea-sized and it's located directly between the two sides of your brain. As part of our body it is directly affected by what we put into that body in the form of food, drink and chemicals of all kinds. As we saw earlier in the book the Pineal Gland is not protected by the "brain-blood-barrier" which inhibits harmful elements flowing directly to our brain. This is part of the reason why the gland is more susceptible to what we eat, drink and ingest than the rest of our brain. While our brain does need some very specific food types, to help it get the energy it needs to function, our Pineal Gland can be the most vulnerable part of the brain when it comes to the wrong kind of diet. In addition to diet there are some chemicals that we routinely ingest and these can be particularly harmful to our Pineal Gland. In this chapter we'll look at the practical steps you can take to de-calcify your Pineal Gland through your diet.

Fluoride and the Pineal Gland

Fluoride is present in our diets in surprisingly large amounts – it's naturally occurring and one of the important minerals we need. However, as with anything in life, it's possible to have too much of a good thing. Our modern diets are fluorinated to a startling extent; fluoride is added to our water, to toothpaste, to sodas, to processed foods and to canned foods. It's everywhere! Unfortunately, this overdose of fluoride means it makes its way to our Pineal Gland and it's one of the major causes of calcification in this part our body. The following steps should be taken to reduce your fluoride intake to a natural amount.

Tap water is usually fluorinated and it's important to avoid this in order to de-calcify your Pineal Gland. Use a water filter or buy purified, distilled water.

Toothpaste is the next big source of overkill on the fluoride front. Increasingly, as we become more concerned about our health in general, it's far easier to buy low fluoride varieties – or better still those with no fluoride at all.

Avoid red meat (occasional amounts are OK and should be part of your diet) and any and all processed foods that you can.

Try to eat only organic fruit and vegetables. The non-organic variety contain a cocktail of drugs and chemicals, many of which are harmful to your health in general.

While some of these steps may be relatively easy, some may take some time to adopt and incorporate into your lifestyle. Persevere until you are, mostly, avoiding the most harmful of these. The benefits will begin to become apparent as your Pineal Gland opens and your Third Eye activates. However, while the psychic benefits are great, the real physical benefits that you'll reap in terms of better health and resistance to illness and infection are worth the effort on their own!

Supplements That Can Help

In addition to foods and products to avoid, there are several dietary supplements that will help to speed the process of de-calcifying your Pineal Gland. These are listed below.

Iodine; supplements containing iodine help to reduce high levels of fluoride in the body. As a supplement this is great for your health, as it moderates the amount of fluoride in your system (we do need some). It can also help to ensure that your de-calcified Pineal Gland is not subject to further deposits.

Tamarind; this food is good for your de-calcification as it helps, as with iodine supplements, to reduce fluoride levels in the body. However, it seems particularly to have an effect on the Pineal Gland, helping to block deposits of calcium.

Cod Liver Oil; good for the body and, it seems, the mind. This product contains high levels of Omega 3, a natural fatty acid, which is important for keeping your joints supple and is also an essential "brain-food". This supplement will ensure a healthy body and a healthy brain, including your Pineal Gland.

Bentonite Clay; this is a good detox supplement which removes chemicals and heavy metals from your system. As the Pineal Gland is more at risk from contamination by these than other parts of the brain it's a great supplement to consider.

Ginseng; again this is a popular detox supplement and can be simply drunk in the form of tea. It helps to remove toxins from the body (benefiting the Pineal Gland) and it also is known to increase the function of the immune system, giving an all-round health boost.

Melatonin; this is the hormone produced by the Pineal Gland itself and it can be severely affected by calcification. Low levels of melatonin can lead to chronic depression, fatigue and anxiety issues. Melatonin supplements will boost your mental state and help to encourage normal function in the Pineal Gland.

Traditional Techniques

In addition to these practical steps that will help you to de-calcify your Pineal Gland, there are a number of alternative methods that you can use. These are based on traditional techniques used in a variety of traditions – some new, some old – to help re-activate or activate the Third Eye. These can be, possibly should be, used in conjunction with the steps above.

Essential Oils; these can be used in your bath, on your pillow or during meditation (more on this later). Essential oils that have been traditionally associated with the Third Eye (Sixth Chakra) are; lavender, pine, frankincense and Davana oil.

Turn off the Lights; the Pineal Gland is sensitive to light and darkness but the latter has been banished from our world almost completely by the widespread use of electric lighting! In fact, lights and screens of all kind mimic natural daylight, which effectively short-circuits our Pineal Gland. Learn to embrace the darkness in your life by turning off gadgets and any non-natural light source from time to time! Ideally, the last hour or so before bed should be natural light only. You can use candles or very low lighting (whichever is safest, most suitable and practical) but be sure to get away from the always-on approach on a daily basis.

Linked to the above, is learning to allow your body to fall asleep and awaken naturally. This will help to re-adjust your natural body-clock which is regulated by the Pineal Gland. In addition to the above tip, practice waking up as it becomes light and allowing your body to gradually come round as it gets lighter.

Chanting "Om" may sound an unlikely way in which to stimulate the Pineal Gland but modern science has discovered that the sound has a direct physical impact on the brain and the skull. It simply creates a real, physical vibration which, although the reasons are unclear as yet, helps to stimulate the Pineal Gland.

Smart phones, or any wireless device emit electro-magnetic waves (EMF). These waves have been found to potentially cause damage to the Pineal Gland (and possibly other parts of the body and brain). Most of us cannot live without these devices today – but try to limit the time you spend with them.

Crystal Healing; another ancient technique and one that has long held associations with the Chakras and re-balancing energy.

In this case any crystal or precious stone colored purple is believed to help heal the Chakra and/or the Pineal Gland. These include purple sapphire, tourmaline and amethyst – though there are many others and choosing your favorite is no bad idea! We'll take a further more detailed look at crystal healing later in this book.

Chapter 6: Types Of Reiki Healing

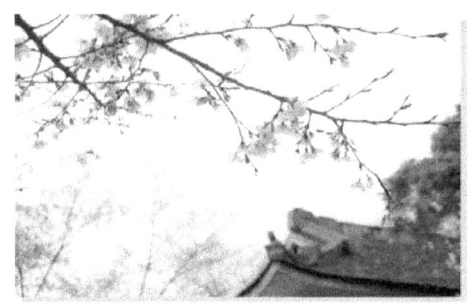

As we discussed previously, there are different types of Reiki that date back years before the Usui Reiki while others are adaptations of Usui Reiki. Each method uses different symbols; however, the principle behind them is the same. In this chapter, you will learn some of the most commonly used Reiki methods.

Usui Reiki

This is considered the first form of Reiki that was brought to the modern world in 1922 by Mikao Usui. It was Hawayo Takata, a Japanese-American born in Hawaii, who brought the Usui Reiki to the West. There have been many changes to the original version of Usui Reiki Ryoho, which is what we know it as now. Usui Reiki differs from how it was taught originally.

Karuna Reiki

Karuna is a Sanskrit word that can be found in the Hinduism, Zen, and Buddhism. This word means compassion. This Reiki healing was created by William Lee Rand, who was the president of The International Center for Reiki Training. This type of Reiki is usually used when trying to relieve the suffering of others. It involves chanting to strengthen the process of healing.

Rainbow Reiki

This type of Reiki was created some time in the 90s by Walter Lübeck, who's a Reiki master in Germany. It is based on the Western teachings of Usui Reiki. With Rainbow Reiki, new techniques have been created such as chakra work, karma clearing, and inner child work.

Kundalini Reiki

Kundalini Reiki focuses on raising healing energy through the first chakra instead of using the crown chakra. Ole Gabrielsen, a Master of Meditation from Denmark, introduced this method. Kundalini is typically practiced with yoga and can get rid of any blockages that your chakras have. It helps to promote greater peace and strengthen.

Choosing the Right Reiki

While the four types of Reiki we just discussed are not the only ones out there, having such a wide variety to choose from can confuse those that are new to this type of healing. So, how do you figure out which Reiki you should use?

Using Usui Reiki is going to appeal to the traditionalists because it is considered to be the original style. However, some say that there are types that have developed since Usui Reiki have improved on healing. There have even been some students of Mikao Usui who made changes to what their teacher invented to create their own style of Reiki.

Every Reiki will have its own parameter regarding the use of symbols, attunements, and levels. A lot of people are confused on which one to pick.

The first thing everyone agrees on is that every form of Reiki uses life force energy. Some people believe that there are greater and lesser forms of life force energy. But, in reality, there are no types of life force energy because it is a free-flowing energy and can be found in all life forms.

One of the easiest ways to visualize life force energy is to visualize water. If you do not have water, you do not have life; and without life force energy, there cannot be life. And just like there are different types of water, the underlying principle is that water provides life to those around it.

Now, remembering that water is water and Reiki is Reiki, you can start to understand that it is not always going to appear that way. For example, you can have a bowl of room-temperature water and in that bowl; you will see different forms take place like the water being frozen or turning into condensation. No matter what form it is in, it is still going to be water.

Just like water, Reiki is around us and it must have a clear channel to flow; and it never runs out. Should a drop of water be evaporated, it becomes a part of the universe again only to come back down to earth. No matter what form it is in, water is always going to be water!

On the other hand, water takes on many different "attitudes". Water can be soft and gentle or it can be a powerful force like a hurricane or a tsunami.

Much the same as water, Reiki goes on forever and has many forms. It can also be experienced as a gentle storm or a powerful force. Since you can experience Reiki in so many different ways, every type

is considered a legitimate way to

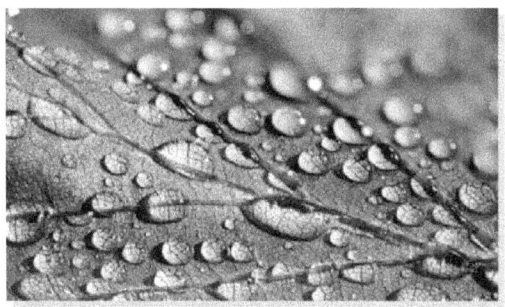

experience the healing it can provide.

You will know what type of Reiki is for you based on the experience you want to have with the energy and what form you are searching for in your life. Take for instance, Reiki may be too powerful for you because you need a gentler approach or you could be looking for something even more powerful.

In the end, you won't make the wrong choice because one is not better than the other. The best way to find the right Reiki for you is to learn about its different types and then allow your intuition to be your guide.

And remember, you can simply speak to a Reiki practitioner so they can help you find the right one for you!

Chapter 7: Understand The Levels Of Reiki

There are certain levels of mastery which you need to understand and its level. You have to know about the entire process before you get Reiki session done. You need to have general understanding of the levels which work the best for you. As the mastery level increases, the levels increases as well. There are three basic levels of Reiki which form the healing and the touch which creates energy in you. You will be able to get the clear understanding and learn a lot from these lessons so get started with learning.

13. The First Degree – Level 1

The practitioners know better about the levels but you can learn them as well and when you go to them you can tell them which level you want. The first level is related to get connected with the universal life and physical life together. The energy forces you to get through the physical being and come out spiritually. By taking the hand down from the head to the hands, it helps you to release the stress by keeping nothing in the mind for some time. You have to concentrate well in order for it to work.

Many people can practice the level 1 by their own as well. people are encouraged to learn it because it is easy and the more you will be able to do it yourself, you can make yourself aware of it and get released from any kind of tension anytime with the help of self-Reiki session. Many people feel the reaction as the heat or coolness in their palms which tells that it is working and they have started to release the tension or stress from their life.

14. Second Degree – Level 2

Now here in level 2, the energy expands and the symbols start to be seen. The more deeply you understand the symbols, the more you will be able to understand your qualities and focus on your present rather than worrying about your future. You can send the positive vibes and the energy can be restored. You cannot reach to level 2 by skipping level 1 so it is important that you have the experience of level 1 and then you can reach level 2. The emphasis of level 2 is to keep the healing process going on. You need to practice on the symbols and have the qualities being identified. You will feel more confident and will tend to respond better to the situations.

15. Third Degree (the Master level) – Level 3

Third degree is also known as mastery level which is considered to be the last level of it. The emphasis of this degree is to make the attunement aligned with the receiving energy. The practitioners make sure to provide the ultimate source of the level 3 mastery of Reiki sessions to the clients. You have to be deeply committed to become a reiki master. If you are a practitioner then make sure you have all the focus and you are free from any negative thought by yourself. The more positive you will be, the more you will be able to relax the other person. You have to concentrate on your work by aiming at providing ease to the other person by giving them the best services. There are many methods through which you can provide the reiki sessions but all of them fall into the levels which have been mentioned. You can choose the right one for you but make sure to follow step by step so that you can master in that.

Chapter 8: The Power Of Attunements

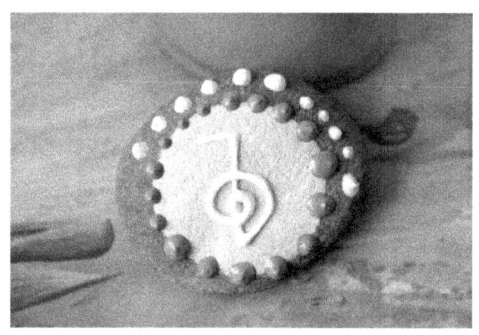

Before you can begin practicing Reiki on yourself and others, you'll need to go through a Reiki Attunement process. Each level of Reiki you learn is going to have additional attunements to open you up to different aspects of Reiki. For example, the Reiki Symbols are part of the Reiki Level II attunement process.

Reiki Attunements are the process in which a Reiki Master opens you up to become a channel for the universal energy. Once you receive an attunement, you are forever going to be a channel for

Reiki energy, however, the way you live your life is going to be a part of keeping yourself a clear and open conduit for Reiki energy.

You can go years without every practicing Reiki and still retain the attunement. Some people who go long periods of time without practicing Reiki might find that they benefit from receiving an attunement to help clear themselves out and reconnect them Reiki energy. It is not necessary, though.

The Reiki Level I attunement is going to be your first step into using Reiki on yourself and others. The Level I attunement ceremony consists of four attunements that each correspond to one of the four degrees of Reiki Level I. The ceremony includes all four Level I attunements that you can receive during your Reiki Level I course, or at the end of your Reiki Level I course.

A Reiki Level II attunement ceremony is the process that opens you up to the Reiki power symbols. There are three symbols that Dr. Usui discovered and that are part of the Reiki Level II attunement ceremony. This ceremony will be slightly different from the Reiki Level I attunement ceremony because it opens you to a different type of Reiki energy.

The attunement ceremony for the Master Level of Reiki is going to attune you to the Master Reiki Symbol. This symbol is not one of the original power symbols that Dr. Usui used and is only attuned during a Master Level attunement ceremony. This Master attunement ceremony also gives you the knowledge and Reiki wisdom to teach and attune students to Reiki Levels as well.

There are additional attunements for advanced Reiki techniques such as for Crystal Reiki and even Reiki for Animals.

The goal of a Reiki attunement is to clear your body, mind, and spirit of any dissonant energy to ensure that you become a clear conduit for Reiki.

Before the Attunement

Prior to receiving any of your attunements, there are some steps you can take to prepare. While the steps of preparation are optional, it will enhance your experience through your studies and also make the attunements more enjoyable and powerful.

In the twenty-four hours before your attunement ceremony, try to avoid any drug use, recreational and pharmaceutical if possible, and alcohol consumption. Any mind-altering substances or medications that change the chemical composition of your mind or body can hide the true beliefs that cause your suffering.

By abstaining from such substances, you can clear the mind and body to be more alert to your own senses, perceptions, and thoughts. This will greatly enhance your attunement ceremonies and make you a more effective conduit for Reiki energy.

Important note: If you are taking prescribed medications by a medical professional for any kind of condition or treatment of a disease or illness, please keep taking those medications unless your doctor or medical professional says it is okay to abstain for twenty-four hours.

Another good step to take for the attunement ceremony is to adjust your diet for the twenty-four hours before an attunement and after an attunement. Try to consume only whole, clean foods in that time. Whole, clean foods include legumes, fresh fruits, and vegetables.

Highly processed foods, chemically altered foods, and foods that are covered in preservatives can create blocks in the channels just like alcohol and drugs. By cleansing the body with clean, whole foods that are raw, unprocessed, and healthy will help open up the energetic channels in your body for the attunement ceremony. By continuing that diet for twenty-four hours after receiving the attunement will help you fully feel the effects of your attunement and your connection to Reiki.

By removing any kind of crutch that the body gains from alcohol, drugs, and unclean foods, you have the opportunity to release the stored energy and beliefs that are fed by and supported by those crutches. Those beliefs, memories, and energy stores don't serve your highest self, so releasing them before an attunement is recommended.

For up to a week prior to your attunement, meditating every day leading up to the attunement ceremony and then every day for a week after the ceremony is also going to be helpful. It is recommended that you make mediation a regular part of your daily routine, and practicing that before and after the attunement ceremony can help you to develop that habit.

This mediation process can help you to make the shifts and changes in your life that you hope to sustain with your study of Reiki. After receiving your attunement, you can include a self-treatment session in with your meditation practice as a part of your daily routine.

Reiki Attunement

A Reiki attunement ceremony is performed by a Reiki Master. The Reiki Master performs a routine that includes the Reiki symbols that were discovered by Dr. Usui. During the ceremony, an intention is set for the highest good of the student, the person receiving the attunement.

The Reiki Master will set an intention to strengthen the student's connection to Reiki energy.

Think of the energies in your body like radio waves or radio stations. By changing the radio station, you can change what information you are receiving, such as news, music, the genre of music, talk shows, etc. Just like you can change a radio station to receive different information, you can retune, or reprogram the body to receive different information, like Reiki energy and wisdom.

Without an attunement ceremony, your body does have access to Reiki energy. Everyone's body has access to Reiki energy. It is a part of the universe and a part of being human. Getting attuned to Reiki energy ensures that you as a student and practitioner receive the proper energy signal for Reiki.

A Reiki attunement ceremony takes about twenty to thirty minutes. As the student or recipient of a Reiki ceremony, all you need to do is find a quiet, relaxed space where you will be undisturbed for the course of the ceremony. Just like when you meditate, you may want to play some calming music, have dim lighting and candles, or burn some incense.

Depending on the type of course you take, you might receive your Reiki attunements in person or from a distance. Both are powerful and acceptable methods for receiving and attunement. If you are taking an in-person class and you receive your attunement from your Reiki Master in person, they may have you sit in a chair so they can move around you with ease during the attunement ceremony.

It is recommended that during a Reiki attunement ceremony, you turn off phones, computers, and find a location that is away from sources of the internet and heavy electronic presences. Since Reiki is energy it can come into conflict with other strong energy sources which come from electronics and the internet. In person attunements are generally performed in complete silence.

Whether you are receiving an attunement in person or from a distance, you may have some interesting experiences, like images and sensations. Some students fall asleep during their attunement ceremonies, this isn't uncommon. Other students don't notice anything at all, just feel relaxed. Everyone experiences attunements differently. There is no right or wrong way to experience a Reiki attunement ceremony.

Some common experiences that people have include are varying sensations like hot, cold, or tingling. You could get visions and see images, or even smell or hear things that are a result of Reiki energy.

Some courses of study will perform attunement ceremonies for all three levels of Reiki at once. Other courses will separate the attunement ceremonies out for each level that the student completes.

As with the experiences you have during your attunement ceremony, there is no right or wrong way to receive them.

Each attunement releases dissonant energy from within you and returns your body, mind, and spirit to a natural energetic frequency that your body wants to remain aligned with.

Receiving a Reiki Level I attunement gives you the basics to treat yourself with Reiki and others with Reiki. It is recommended that go through at least Reiki Level II if you'd like to work on clients or recipients, especially in a professional setting.

Going through the Reiki Level II attunement ceremony and the Reiki Master attunement ceremony your body will draw in yet another kind of Reiki energy which is what attunes you to the Reiki symbols and gives you the wisdom to perform attunement ceremonies.

During a ceremony, nothing is actually shifting in your mind, body or spirit. Rather Reiki provides you with a guidance down a path to make shifts that serve your highest good. Your body begins to release, but it is in the inclusion of daily self-treatments after your attunements that push the healing forward and continue to aid you.

Most people that are interested in learning Reiki are ready to release and heal by the time they make the commitment to become a Reiki student. The practice of separating the attunements out was traditionally used in order to ensure that a student was committed to going through each level without rushing the process.

Rushing the attunement ceremonies can result in the student not learning or practicing to the full extent of each level before moving on. Additionally, some students might go through one attunement and then decide that Reiki is for them.

There are times when the energetic shifts happen after an attunement almost immediately. Other times the shifts can take time, practice, and study to occur. The mind puts limitations on itself, especially if you hear a limitation aloud. If a Reiki Master says 'You can't handle more than one Reiki Level Attunement at once,' then the mind imposes that limitation. However, there is no evidence to suggest that attunements can't be performed in one ceremony.

Whatever the case, you should look for a Master who offers the attunement ceremonies in the way that you wish to receive them.

After the Attunement

It isn't uncommon to feel the flow of Reiki energy through your body immediately following an attunement ceremony. If you don't sense energy right away, that is okay. That doesn't mean there is something wrong with you. It doesn't mean that the attunement didn't work.

Your body is only able to perceive a fraction of energy at any given time, yet the universe is full of energy and anything made of matter is made of energy. It can take time for your body to adjust its perception of Reiki energy.

Your body may begin to change in other ways. Your hands might feel warmer, or tingle and emanate energy when you are around people that are in need of Reiki energy. You'll have to learn to adjust to these sensations. Overtime, you may experience different sensations or shifts in the energy.

If any of the sensations are uncomfortable or overwhelming, take a few deep breaths and set an intention in your mind to allow the Reiki to flow freely through you. This will help release the buildup of intense energy. With practice on yourself, you will begin to learn how to channel the flow of energy and when and how to restrict the flow.

Your body, mind, and spirit will begin to release energy and clear energy. Imbalances will start to be brought back into alignment. Stagnation starts to move and flow again. Any energies that are no longer serving your highest good are transmuted and shifted. These shifts are important to your personal healing, but also to your ability to channel Reiki energy at the highest frequency.

In order to heal, your body must be clear of imbalances. Energetic imbalances are what create dis-ease and lead to the manifestation of physical, emotional, and mental symptoms. After a Reiki attunement ceremony, your body has the wisdom to heal itself. Continuing to promote energy shifts and keeping yourself a clear conduit is what is going to make the largest impact on your personal healing and the raising of your energetic vibration.

You might want to keep track of any changes that you notice occurring. Sometimes having a documented progression of shifts and changes can really help you understand how you are benefitting. If you'd like to use Reiki as a service to help heal others, providing them with personal experiences can help on their road to healing as well.

Once you are attuned to Reiki, it is very important to perform daily self-treatments of Reiki. This is going to keep your body open to Reiki energy and guidance as well as continue to correct any imbalances in your body. Those imbalances will then extend outward into your environment and the lifestyle you live. It is also the best way to keep your body infused with Reiki energy for long-term success and fulfilment.

Drinking adequate amounts of water and keeping your diet as whole and clean as possible are also methods that will help you gain more sensitivity and awareness to energies around you. These are also health practices that will only contribute to your overall health and wellness.

Since Reiki is intuitive, you will need to trust Reiki to heal what needs to be healed. As you perform self-treatments you will begin to understand what this means. That is another reason it is so important to keep up with daily self-treatments once you are attuned.

Reiki Attunements are the ceremonies that are going to open you up to the healing power of Reiki, the wisdom of the universe, and the guiding hand of Reiki energy. When you are ready to receive your attunements and go through the Reiki Level I course, if you have not already done so, be sure to find a Reiki Master that you resonate with and feel like you can learn from.

When you are working closely with someone who is going to be tuning your energy frequencies and guiding you on the attunement journey, you'll want someone you trust. You'll want a Reiki Master that can answer your questions, isn't too busy to make time for their students outside of their set courses, and someone who understands your goals with learning Reiki. Having the right Reiki Master to perform your attunement ceremonies is just as important to your healing journey.

Attunement ceremonies should be enjoyable. It is rare that anyone doesn't enjoy the attunement ceremony, but go into the ceremony with an open mind and no expectations.

Chapter 9: Healing Others & Animals

After you have gone through the process of healing on yourself enough times you should start to feel confident enough to use Reiki to heal others. Allow the healing process to feel natural and be confident in the fact that you have been working with this energy and it can work for others. The best way to start healing others is to begin with family members and friends who are willing to try Reiki healing. Even if those who are close to you, don't feel sick, assure them that at the very least the process of Reiki healing can help them to feel relaxed and give them an overall feeling of well being. However, beyond that you should never promise specific results from a healing sitting. The process of healing is unique to every person and can be an unknown depending on what is wrong with someone. Let your volunteer know what Reiki can do and assure them that they will see some benefit as everyone does.

Another great thing about beginning to heal others beside yourself is that while you are giving healing to someone else you get a benefit as well. The more you work with Reiki energy and the more sittings that you do, the better your natural balance with the energy is, the more balanced you feel the more you can work with the energy so it benefits everyone.

The hand positions you will use on others are the same as the ones you use on yourself with one added:

Position 1: Run your hands over the entire body just above it not actually touching, checking for hot spots in the energy.

Position 2: Link your hands together on the top of the subject's head

Position 2: Place one hand on the subject's forehead, then place the other at the back of their neck about one hand length above the base of your neck.

Position 3: Place your hands gently over the subject's eyes

Position 4: Place your hands gently over the subject's ears

Position 5: Place one hand on the subject's upper torso and place the other on your rib cage.

Position 6: Place your hands on the subjects hips

Before you begin a session with someone briefly go over the hand positions with them. It is important for them to feel relaxed and comfortable before you lay hands on them and knowing where your hands may go will aid in that.

Once you have gone over the hand positions the best position to ask your subject to take for the healing is laying down. Give them a comfortable area on a table, bed or the floor with their head supported so that you can easily reach the back of their neck. Playing some music and having incense or candles can also help the subject relax and prepare to feel the healing wash over them.

Once they are laying you will perform your beginning hand positions with the intent to heal. As you should be familiar with by now you will be gracious to the energy and asking for it to help. Then you will follow your instincts and go through the positions of the hands to find the spots on your subject that need healing. It is often best to start with position one and do a full scan of the energy around the person. This allows your senses to stretch and easily pinpoint the hot spots for them that will need your help. As with self healing the amount of time a session will take can vary on your subject. Listen to your instincts and follow your balance and harmony with the energy. Once you have completed the healing you will again thank the energy that helped you and allow it to go back to normal flow.

While not required, having a subject remain lying down for 5-10 minutes after a healing can be beneficial to keep them relaxed, especially if they are a first time recipient of Reiki. You can also take this time to gently ask what they did or did not feel during the process. Some will report tingling, sensations of colors and a variety of other things, though others will report they felt nothing. That doesn't mean the healing did not work and you will want to assure them of that the experience is simply different for everyone.

Don't feel disappointed if the first times you think there is no noticeable effect with the healing you have given. Sometimes it just takes a little longer or more then one session to show. If someone has a long history of deep emotional issues, it can be harder for them to let them go all at once and while the energy aids in this, it can sometimes take more than one session or just a longtime to truly begin to show results. Just as with open wounds or surgery everyone's healing process is different. Trust in the process and the Reiki.

Healing Animals

Many of us have animals that we do not just see as pets but family members and we always want to do the best we can for them. They are living and they do have energy about them so Reiki can benefit and heal them as well as humans. Reiki can help illness, pain, anxiety and behavior issues in your pets. The important thing to remember when you treat your animals is that they are a little different than us, the intent to heal will be the same but the laying of hands for them is different.

Rather the specific hand placements allow your instincts to guide you to where they need help. If it is a physical illness or injury you will likely already know one place to go but behavior issues can be many different places. You will lay your hands gently where you are guided. If the pet is a little fidgety and doesn't want to sit perfectly still that is okay, do not force it simply make sure you keep your hands within 4 inches of the affected area, Reiki will still flow if your hands are off the body but remain within 4 inches. From here the process is the exact same as a human, stay in the place as long as you need to and dismiss the energy politely when done.

Reiki is a great healer and many have found it to be beneficial to their furry loved ones who have been through trauma in the past be they rescues or a tragic accident that happened and changed their personality. Reiki is the perfect way to return every member of your family back to perfect health.

Chapter 10: Angel Jar

I got this idea to make this Angel Jar from Angels. While reading angel cards for myself, I got this "GOD BOX" card. Somehow I ignored the message and did not make this God Box. I started getting this GOD BOX card whenever I used to do angel reading for myself. So one fine day, I decided to make God Box. I looked around in the house but could not come up with any box that would give the feeling of perfect box. Then out of blue, a plastic jar caught my eye. That was IT. I painted and decorated the jar. Left in the balcony for the paint to dry. Later, I saw a beautiful butterfly hovering over my jar. Hence the name 'Angel Jar'.

You can use any box or jar. Name it God Box, Angel Box, Angel Jar or even fairy box. Basically the concept of this 'Angel Jar' or 'God Box' is to handover/transfer all your worries to higher authorities.

- Take a Box or a Jar. Decorate it if you want to.
- Pray and call upon God, Angels, Ascended Masters, Guides or Faeries. Tell them that you are giving away all your fears to them to deal with it.
- On a paper write down all your worries, troubles, doubts, fears or whatever is troubling you in details. Write as if you are sharing your problem with someone.
- **Draw whatever reiki symbols you are attuned to on the back side of the paper. Give reiki to this paper with the intention that** you are now depositing all your worries, fears and problems into this jar and you are letting your angels take care of those issues.
- Important☐ Trust that it is taken care of now.
- Do not re-read your slips often. Read out loud after 15-20 days and burn these slips. Write fresh ones with new or old issues. You can decorate the slips if you want to or you can keep it simple. Totally up to

you. Do not hesitate to write any problem. Pen down any issue big or small. Be sure that it will be taken care of now. It is not a magic box so keep your expectations in control☐

Crystal Water for Healing

All crystals and gemstones have different properties and unique abilities to heal. I am not writing about crystal healing and laying of stones. Today I am writing about Healing with Crystal Water/Essence. Few days back, during wee hours, I was in deep sleep and out of nowhere I heard CRYSTAL WATER in my mind. I was confused as where this thought popped from. I took it as a sign from angels. So later during the day, I started looking up on internet about it. And Bingo! I found lots many wonderful technique for healing. I tried simplest one to make Crystal Water. So far I have made Rose quartz water, citrine water and clear quartz water. Crystal essence or crystal water has been used for healing purpose since ages. They can be made easily and can be stored to re-use. There are many ways to make Crystal Water. Some add vodka or vinegar as preservatives. I prefer making it simpler way as I do not prefer preservatives. The crystal water made without preservatives may last up to 20 days. Make sure that you do not use just any crystal as some crystals may have toxic components. **Study crystal properties before using them.**

• Choose the crystal or crystals according to your issue. Suppose if you want to make money essence use citrine or if you want for love you can use rose quartz.

• Ground yourself. Stay calm and relaxed. Do some prayer or meditation.

• Cleanse your crystal. Hold it in your palm. Invoke angel's help, ask your crystals for help. Draw reiki symbols and infuse the flow of reiki. State your intention and give reiki to your crystal for about 5-10 minutes. Hold your intention while charging your crystal with reiki. To heal others, dedicate the symbol to someone by stating their name 3 times along with intention.

• Now here we have 2 ways to make crystal water-

(1) Take 2 glass containers. One big and one small. Put your reiki infused crystal in small container and if possible close the container.

Fill big container with spring water or filtered water. Place the small container with crystal in the big container. Take care that the container with crystal doesn't topple. Put the containers out in sunlight or moon light for 4-5 hours. Your crystal water is ready.

(2) Another is way simpler method. Put your reiki infused crystal directly in a glass container filled with spring water or filtered water. Leave your container in sunlight or moon light for few hours. Your crystal water is ready.

• When your crystal water is half consumed, you can add more water to it

and again leave it in sunlight or moon light.

Additionally, you can place extra crystals pointed towards container around the container.

Alternatively, you let sit crystals in water for 24 hours and then use it.

Once every 15-20 days cleanse your container, crystals and do above process to refill and recharge.

Fill this water in dark colored bottle like cobalt blue or green.

The more crystals you put, the stronger the crystal water is.

Mix 5-6 drops of crystal water with drinking water to consume.

When consuming this water, make sure that crystals stays in container and doesn't drop in your glass.

You can carry this water to school, office or wherever you go, to keep you charged with crystal healing.

You can water your plants with Crystal water, with 3-4 drops of crystal water added to one glass of water.

It is safe for pets too. Add 3-4 drops of crystal water to one bowl of water.

Fill in spray bottle and spray on yourself or affected person.

Remove negativity from home or work space by spraying crystal water.

Can be applied directly to skin.

Crystal Water is also known as: Crystal elixirs, gem elixirs, gem waters, crystal tonics, gem tonics, gem essences, crystal essence and more.

If you decide to use more than one type of crystal, make sure the properties of crystals are same. Try not make 'crystal chaos' by adding too many.

Double check crystals properties before putting in water as some are **HIGHLY TOXIC**. For 'risky' stones always use Method 1.

Be innovative and make use of crystal water as much as you can☐

Chi-Ball the chakras

Chakra cleansing is the key to a healthy and happy life. Unbalanced or blocked chakras may create havoc on physical as well as emotional level. Every healer has their own way of chakra cleansing. Below is a method using energy ball/ chi ball for chakra cleansing.

First thing I always do before activating reiki flow is invoking Angels, guides, Gods and ascended masters to bless me with their presence and help me with healing.

Crown Chakra- Activate reiki and draw reiki symbols on your palm. Start making an energy ball/chi ball. Visualize the chi ball of the color of crown chakra that is Violet. Imagine reiki symbols floating in the violet ball. Chant symbol names thrice. State your intent to cleanse, clear and unblock your crown chakra. Say crown chakra affirmation thrice- I connect easily with Divine wisdom. Release the chi ball.

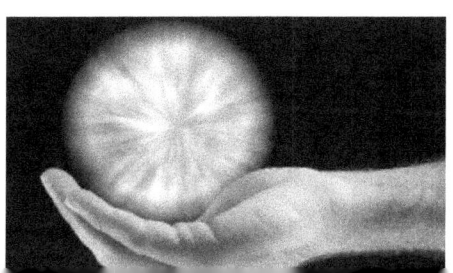

Brow Chakra- Make another chi ball. Visualize the chi ball of the color of brow chakra that is Indigo/dark blue. Imagine reiki symbols floating in the indigo ball. Chant symbol names thrice. State your intent to cleanse, clear and unblock your brow chakra. Say brow chakra affirmation thrice- I fully and totally trust my intuition. Release the chi ball.

Throat Chakra- Make another chi ball. Visualize the chi ball of the color of throat chakra that is Blue. Imagine reiki symbols floating in the blue ball. Chant symbol names thrice. State your intent to cleanse, clear and unblock your throat chakra. Say throat chakra affirmation thrice- I express myself with confidence. Release the chi ball.

Heart Chakra- Make another chi ball. Visualize the chi ball of the color of heart chakra that is Green. Imagine reiki symbols floating in the green ball. Chant symbol names thrice. State your intent to cleanse, clear and unblock your heart chakra. Say heart chakra affirmation thrice- I love and accept myself completely. Release the chi ball.

Solar Plexus Chakra- Make another chi ball. Visualize the chi ball of the color of Solar Plexus chakra that is Yellow. Imagine reiki symbols floating in the yellow ball. Chant symbol names thrice. State your intent to cleanse, clear and unblock your solar-plexus chakra. Say solar-plexus chakra affirmation thrice- I manifest my desires easily. Release the chi ball.

Sacral Chakra- Make another chi ball. Visualize the chi ball of the color of Sacral chakra that is Orange. Imagine reiki symbols floating in the orange ball. Chant symbol names thrice. State your intent to cleanse, clear and unblock your sacral chakra. Say sacral chakra affirmation thrice- I easily accept my desires and pleasures. Release the chi ball.

Root Chakra- Make another chi ball. Visualize the chi ball of the color of root chakra that is Red. Imagine reiki symbols floating in the red ball. Chant symbol names thrice. State your intent to cleanse, clear and unblock your root chakra. Say root chakra affirmation thrice- I am safe and loved. Release the chi ball.

Thank your guides and angles.

For distant healing, take a substitute such as a doll or a soft toy. Connect HSZSN to the doll/soft toy. Do above procedure. Release chi ball on each chakra.

Quick Fix- If you are in a hurry and have no time for full procedure, just make a single chi ball, add symbols, put intention to cleanse, clear and unblock all the chakras and release the chi ball.

As I said earlier, chi ball is my personal favorite☐

Chapter 11: Benefits From Increased Reiki Efforts

Once you have a good understanding of Reiki and have begun regular practice, there are a number of other ways to enhance your results. This chapter will go over the many techniques that can be used in conjunction with Reiki to help you to reap maximum results.

Technique #1: Increasing Your Vibration

Your vibrational energy is used to describe the specific energy that you give off. This type of energy varies from person to person and can be affected by a number of factors. That being said, there are several ways that you can go about raising your vibration, including:

Sleeping adequately (an adequate amount is 7-8 hours on average, though some people need more for their body to function well)

Improve your nutritional habits by eating wholesome foods instead of those full of processed ingredients, food dye, and chemicals

Participate in social activities and outings (especially those involving exercise, going outdoors, and nature)

Massage

Yoga and stretching

Meditation

Reiki practice with others

Technique #2: Bring Repressed Fears and Anxieties to the Surface

One of the ways to use Reiki energy to balance fears, anxieties, and other difficulties is to help Reiki balance the fears. After your session, take a minute or two to feel the Reiki flowing through your body. Then, think about what is making you scared or anxious. Feel the power of the Reiki as it flows through your body and combats your fears and anxieties. Remain focused and keep the Reiki feeling until you feel balanced and completely at peace once again.

Technique #3: Reflect on Your Reiki Session Once It Has Ended

Instead of getting to your feet and going about your day as soon as the final timer ding sounds, lie there an additional five minutes and focus on the challenges you are facing in life. If the Reiki session has been successful, then you may find yourself looking at these challenges in new ways. In some cases, you will find a new positive view of the situation. In others, you may find a solution.

Pay close attention to your thoughts and feelings. If you choose, after the reflection, write what you thought of in a journal. You will be able to use this for guidance and reflection on your personal development journey with Reiki.

Technique #4: Repeating Positive Affirmations

If you have ever read a self-help book, then you know the amount of power that can come with the right thoughts. The way that you think really does have the power to change your life. This is true with Reiki as well. Consider whatever your largest goal is for Reiki. This may be pain management for your condition or learning to express yourself in a positive way at work. Write down this goal on a note card that you can carry with you throughout your day. If you choose, you can look up Reiki symbols online and draw these onto the card as well.

When you find yourself thinking about it, read the affirmation on your card. Then, give thanks that your affirmation is coming true. If you wanted more confidence at work, for example, you may say "Thank you for the positive energy that has allowed me to become more confident at work." Do this until you will your wants and desires into existence.

Chapter 12: Reiki Level 2

Reiki Level 2 is available to those who have already received the first level from a properly trained teacher. This module implies a new energy tuning, and it is mandatory for the student to successfully use the new knowledge.

Experience shows that there is no problem that the student receives, in a short period of time, levels 1 and 2, leaving the student subject only to a more intense cleaning process in the subsequent twenty-one days. It is at the discretion of the student the decision on the time that must elapse between the two tunings.

Level 2 is an essential degree for those who not only train themselves to participate in healing but also wish to rescue their divine abilities and obtain the transcendence of imperfect and limited states.

With the new initiation, vast horizons will open before the student, and the spectrum of his psychic faculties will increase considerably, leading him to new spiritual stages. The Reikiano becomes a bridge of union with all the living consciences of the planet and the cosmos, interaction that will allow us to maintain the flow of energy, even in extremely adverse conditions.

The new modality of healing is a unique process that will allow the healing agent to take the patient to a level where the perception of the latter can carry out the transformation of karma, promoting positive changes that reach up to the DNA chains. The initial process of "awakening" evolves toward the path of "transformation," and the therapist goes on to transform the whole, rescuing his condition of well-being and peace. It extrapolates the condition of treating just "that body" or "that condition." He goes on to treat all current bodies and conditions, acting on immortal man.

The Reikiano advances, in turn, from a simple attitude of knowledge to an intervention, without limits, in his conscience, and in the world. The therapist becomes a source in the continuous movement of the maintenance of the divine state. The ability of the Reikian to heal is greatly expanded and intensified. It will be able to purify the energy of any space and environment, quickly.

Level 2 operates mainly on the emotional and mental levels, while the healing in the first module focused mainly on the physical body. The action of energy will happen, first, in the subtle bodies of the person involved. It is understood that the vital energy of the universe is not limited to working only on a plane and in a linear manner, but rather, it seeks the cause of the problem, where it is found, healing the individual irreversibly.

At this level, the student exercises to access the patient's unconscious. We enter a new dimension of healing, which will allow you to heal yourself or others, transforming old negative behaviors into new constructive behaviors. Depressions with emotional origins become transformed, as well as mental disorders, destructure, obsessions, phobias, vices, nervous exhaustion, and tendencies acquired in the mother's womb or in previous lives. We learn to influence our thoughts in a positive way, to recreate and modify them for the better.

The main element of level 2 is the healing, at a distance, of absent people. The Reikian can send divine energy to any place, regardless of space and time. The loving healing energy of Reiki can be sent from this module as if it were a "bridge of light" or an "energy arrow" that fully reaches a previously determined point.

In the energy initiation of level 2, the student is tuned to the frequency of three cosmic Reiki symbols. Learning to work with them will get to direct the energy beyond the physical plane. It will acquire the ability to manage to direct universal, expanded energy, beyond any consideration of time and space.

Chapter 13: Heal Chakṛas And Realign Your Entire Chakra System

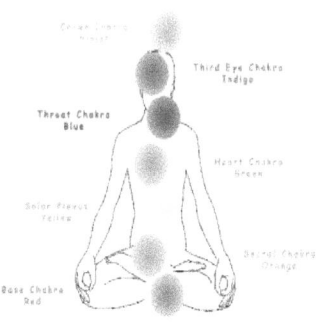

Now that we have connected physical and emotional problems to our specific chakras, it is time to get them back in alignment, so that our body and mind may function properly together. Perhaps you relate to symptoms of the imbalance of one or two specific chakras. While it may be necessary to focus energy on these to realign yourself, we must not forget to look at the big picture. Focusing energy on one chakra inadvertently removes energy from others. We must look at the system as a whole, making sure that every chakra is in the balance, so that we can live a fulfilling, happy life.

Let us start by working on each individual chakra. First, the root, number one. As we discussed, this is the chakra that makes us feel grounded and secure in life. When out of balance, we may have issues with money, we may feel a bit paranoid and unsure of our standing. This chakra is associated with the color red, so, therefore, we may strengthen this chakra with more exposure. It can help to surround ourselves with red things, but it may be more appropriate to eat foods that are red, rather than repainting an entire room.

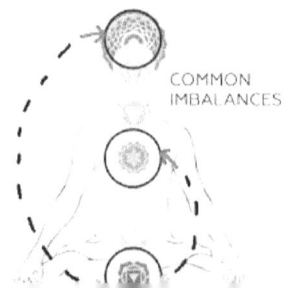

COMMON IMBALANCES

Eat foods that are deep red, like red meat, apples, beets, and red peppers. The color red is also associated with heat and warmth, so foods that are spicy, like hot peppers (red ones), can be beneficial as well. As this is the chakra of grounding, eating foods that come from the ground, like carrots and potatoes, so called 'root vegetables' are beneficial as well.

Certain yoga poses, like the bridge, which stretch muscles and tendons in this area can help move energy around in this area, stimulating the chakra. The action of simply walking barefoot on the earth may help as well. As the idea is grounding, it makes sense to get as close to the earth as possible to accept some new energy.

The second chakra, the sacral, is primarily responsible for connection with others, sexuality, and well-being. It may manifest itself as infertility, low sexual drive, and inability to fully connect with loved ones. Again, we can use food to help heal the chakra. Orange is the associated color, so orange peppers, carrots, and pumpkin are great foods to include.

In yoga, doing exercises like the cobra pose, or pelvic movements can help stretch and unblock energy channels in this area. Any stretches or movements that engage the pelvic area, including belly dancing, can help stimulate sex drive and increase fertility.

The solar plexus chakra is in the upper abdomen, so it would make sense that any movement involving this area would be beneficial. When this chakra is out of alignment, we may feel out of control of our life, and confidence wanes. Doing sit ups and other exercises that engage the core are beneficial. In yoga, doing poses like the boat pose engage the core, or dancing and shaking the hips engages the core as well.

The solar plexus is associated with the color yellow, and so foods that are yellow may help engage the chakra as well. Add lemon to water, and enjoy corn on the cob in the summer. Grains are also beneficial, as well as herbal teas like mint.

The heart chakra must constantly be nourished. Without it, we are not able to love or feel compassion for others. Physically, we may have heart trouble or problems with breathing. Reconnecting to this chakra will be very beneficial to our entire life. The only way to exercise our heart is to use it. In the physical sense, doing cardiovascular exercises like walking or jogging work the heart and lungs. In an emotional sense, we must practice loving and accepting others whole heartedly to exercise our chakra.

While you would expect its associated color to be red, it is actually green. Surrounding yourself with greenery in nature, and eating greens on the regular are great ways to engage your heart chakra. Ever notice how a hike in the woods really enhances your spirit? The combination of exercise and lush green environment stimulate your heart chakra. Eat a big salad and sip on some green tea after a long walk to get your heart in the right place.

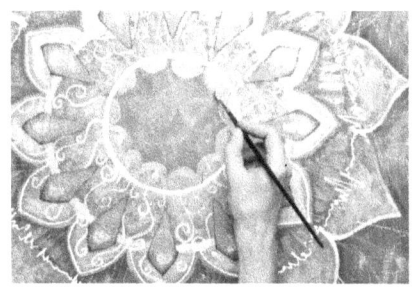

The throat chakra is responsible for effective communication, first and foremost. It also holds the key to the thyroid gland, which makes hormones responsible for energy levels and much more. Imbalances lead to deficits in the thyroid gland, leaving you sluggish and listless. In this state, it will be much more difficult to communicate effectively.

The throat chakra is blue, so eating foods that are rich and blue, like blueberries are your best bet, although any fruit will do. Medically speaking, a person with underactive thyroid should avoid dark green foods, as their properties actually inhibit the thyroid. Do not avoid them altogether, as this can then throw off your heart chakra. Balance is the key here. Exercises that work the shoulders and arms are good for this chakra as well. Doing pushups during a workout and stretching your shoulders out across your chest as you cool down is very stimulating.

Since our third eye chakra provides a deep connection with our spiritual being, we must exercise and connect with it regularly. As it is located between our eyes, there aren't too many traditional exercises that reach this area. Eye motions, like eye rolls (not at your spouse), can work the area, and yoga poses like child's pose that places the forehead on the floor can stimulate it. Connecting with it on a daily basis by listening to cues given by your inner self is helpful as well. The third eye is indigo, and eating purplish blue foods like dark berries are beneficial. Your third eye also likes chocolate and lavender, which explains the need for both during stressful situations.

Finally, our crown chakra, responsible for our greatest spiritual connection, must be fostered. Located at the top of our head, we must get creative to exercise it properly. If you aren't feeling quite right, and are just unable to feel happy, spend some time nurturing the crown chakra. As this is very much mind-related, we must practice meditation and mindfulness to exercise this chakra. It is associated with the color violet, but eating a plethora of violet foods, which there are not many of, isn't overly beneficial. Focus more on your body-spirit connection to keep this chakra healthy.

You will have noticed that aligning all of these chakras has three main components. These are food, which provides energy, exercise, with expends energy, and mind, which balances energy are all required. It only makes sense then, to exercise a host of these three components on a daily basis

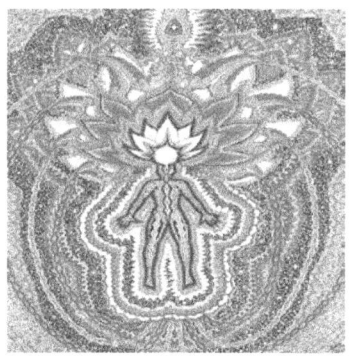

to maintain a powerful chakra system.

You will have noticed that all of the foods mentioned were of good quality and nutrition. We discussed vegetables, fruits, meats, and herbs. No junk food, soda or fast food. This is not by accident. By incorporating foods that come right from the earth, our natural habitat, we are promoting good health of all chakras. Get a wide variety of fruits and veggies of different colors to receive different types of nutrients and energies that the body needs. Combine that with simple proteins from meats, nuts, and seeds for muscle maintenance and proteins that help make up the brain. Dietary fat is important as well, especially oils from olives, avocado, and fish, as the Omega 3 fatty acids within the help support optimal brain function.

A combination of different exercises is important as well. For good health, we must combine moderate intensity exercise like jogging and hiking to promote the heart, circulatory system, and respiratory system. We must also pair this with meaningful stretching to release tension from muscles and target the core and shoulders. Yoga and simple stretching after cardio can help us accomplish this. Remember that our physical body is where our spirit lives. It would be wise to treat it with the utmost respect and care while we are still here.

That said, we must also exercise our mind, mainly for our third eye and crown chakras. As both are centered on the head, the house for our brain, we must remember to use our brains to think logically and tap into the wants and needs of our inner spirit. Ignoring these signals causes our brain to fall into disrepair, and over stresses it. Paying attention to the proper signals leads us to better decision making, and allows us to flow with our natural course of energy.

If you feel that a certain chakra needs attention based on the current course of your life, or if you feel like you need to enhance certain aspects of your life, go ahead and focus some attention on one. Just don't forget that the entire system is connected and neglecting the rest for the sake of one chakra will only bring bigger problems. Do your due diligence to look at the big picture and live a life in balance with your chakra system.

Chapter 14: Reiki Symbols

First Degree Reiki Channel

Once you become a First Degree Reiki Channel through your well-earned First Degree, you become endowed with the ability to heal your body. It is a great experience; and so beneficial! However, apart from you own self there may be other factors in your life that may need healing. You may not be aware of it, but there may be around you areas and segments that require healing. There may be an arduous situation that requires healing. In such a case how do you proceed? A situation is something we find ourselves in. We cannot see it; we can only feel it. How then can we lay on a healing Reiki hand on a situation? And yet we can heal a tight situation and solve difficult problems.

Second Degree Reiki Channel

To be capable of healing matters and concerns of a higher order in your life, you need to move up and graduate into the Second Degree of Reiki. During this course, you will be taught how to use Reiki to heal but without laying on hands. The Second Degree of Reiki will introduce to you the phenomenal Reiki Symbols. Reiki Symbols help the Reiki Channels to send Positive Energy to any situation—any condition—in your life which needs your immediate attention. As a Second Degree of Reiki Channel you can heal other people's predicaments and roadblock too, whether they are material or spiritual.

Before understanding Reiki Symbols, it is important to comprehend the meaning of the word 'symbol'. Symbol comes from the Latin word Symbolium, which is derived from the Greek word Sun Ballein, the meaning of which is throwing, gathering or joining together. Symbols consist mostly of graphic designs or alphabets. For example, the Pentacle (originating in King Solomon's times), the Christian Cross (one of the most ancient human symbols used by many religions) or the Hindu Om which is not only a spiritual symbol but also a mantra and sacred sound in Hinduism, Buddhism and Jainism.

All established symbols generate their own Energy. Whether one is familiar to the symbol or not, merely looking at them will evoke vibrations to your energetic system.

This is exactly what the Reiki Symbol also does. Reiki symbols create a sort of cosmic ladder for Reiki Practitioners to be able to reach an otherwise inaccessible path to attain their objective. It is like a key to the door of the Universe with which Reiki Practitioners can access and obtain whatever they need from the Universe to accentuate and energize their healing process.

Like other sanctified symbols of the world, Reiki Symbols are also sacred. Dr Usui goes a step further to say that Reiki Symbols are also Secret. The Usui System of Reiki advises, as a word to the wise, that a novice should not look upon Reiki Symbols before they are truly attuned to Reiki through the proper conduit. This is also the reason why this book, unlike so many out there on the market, has not included the Reiki Symbols which, according to the Usui System of Reiki, should be looked at and learnt after one gets attuned and initiated by their Reiki Teacher. When the student becomes familiar with the Reiki Symbols, they can then use them for own benefits and for those of the others. Learning about the Reiki Symbols without passing through the proper channel will bring no result to the learner. This is why I believe that sharing images of Reiki Symbols with the un-initiated and the neophytes through books and on the Internet defies the very purpose of Dr Usui's principle of keeping Reiki symbols secret and using them to their utmost usage.

But we can, of course, learn about the Reiki Symbols to be able to get acquainted with their wondrous powers.

It goes without saying that all consecrated symbols should be used correctly. Using them incorrectly can bring in 'incorrect' or erroneous results. For example, some symbols, used in their reversed form (let's say placed upside down) will without doubt become recipients of negative energy. A good example of this is the Pentacle which is a five point star. Placed in the right way—one point up and two points down—it is a positive symbol, representing the Human and everything connected to humanity. The Pentacles' upper point represents the head, the 2 points down symbolize the legs and the side points stand for the arms. The Pentacle is widely used for healing and for other positive energy workings. But when the same symbol is placed or used incorrectly (let's say upside down), it then epitomizes negativity in all its aspects. It is also said that an upside down Pentacle is a sign of Evil. I cited the above example here for the simple reason that any sacred symbol, used outside their accepted norms or incorrectly, can/will become erroneous.

Can One Cause Harm Through Reiki?

This world is not made up of good only. While our planet includes people who do what they know is 'right', there is also a handful of such individuals out there who daily wish harm on others. Many of such people also believe they can use Dr Usui's Reiki Symbols (in a reversed way) to cause harm. Some even go to the extent of pretending that this is true. My answer to such baseless and meritless claims is that they are baseless and devoid of any truth. REIKI SYMBOLS ARE AND WILL REMAIN HEALING SYMBOLS. They can never be used otherwise, try as one may. Dr Usui's rationale during all his lifetime was to make humans take charge of their own existence, to work honestly and to bring in positive results in all aspects of their lives. How could a large-hearted and philanthropic man like Dr Usui even think of putting dangerous and harmful tools in the hands of man? I believe that using Reiki Symbols for any other purpose than nursing one back to health and happiness is a useless try out which can only cause harm to the one trying to achieve it. Reiki Symbols, learnt and used in the approved manner will bring only positive results. If used otherwise it simply will not work.

The 3 Wonderful Reiki Symbols

When you go for Reiki attunement through your Second Degree of Reiki, you will be attuned to 3 wonderful Reiki Symbols. They are as follows:

Cho Koo Ray - the Power Symbol

Meaning: Bring the Power Here (as translated by Master Takata)

The Reiki Symbol Cho Koo Ray is a true Energy amplifier. It is of vital importance to increase the flow of Reiki for both the Giver and the Receiver of Reiki. The Reiki Symbol Cho Koo Ray is used for protection, for cleansing the atmosphere of negative energies and also for self healing and for healing others.

Sei Hei Ki: the Mental/Emotional Symbol

Meaning: God and Humanity Come Together

The meaning of the Reiki Symbol Sei Hei Ki is understandable. It specifies that when one suffers, for example mentally or emotionally, experiencing agitations like the loss of a loved one, loneliness or poverty, the Reiki Symbol Sei Hei Ki helps in a divine way to alleviate pain and to soothe the human mind and body. Sei Hei Ki heals and brings respite in all agonizing situations and relationships. Reiki Symbol Sei Hei Ki is also used for finding misplaced/lost things, for memorizing and for remembrance. This prodigious Symbol is also used for healing animals, whether pets or not.

Hon Sha Ze Sho Nen: The Distant or Absent Symbol

Meaning: The God in Me Meets the God in You

The Reiki Symbol Hon Sha Ze Sho Nen helps heal a patient even in his or her absence. This amazing symbol is also used for personal empowerment, for healing past painful incidents which hold back or get in the way of one's present, for sending Reiki Healing to future events and also for achieving goals.

All the three Reiki Symbols mentioned above are used to intensify the flow of Reiki Energy. Reiki Channels should take note that the more Reiki they do on themselves and on others, the more Energy will flow through their hands and will become stronger with time and practice. They will also find it easier to get rid or let go of all that is not required in their life.

I remind readers once again that Reiki symbols in themselves and all the information that can be obtained about them are of little or no value on their own. It is mandatory for all those who want to learn about the Reiki symbols that they undergo Reiki initiation through an established Reiki Master.

As the Second Degree Reiki Channels move on to the Third Degree of Reiki, they will become acquainted with the fourth Reiki Symbol.

Dai Koo Myo: The Master Symbol

Meaning: O Great Beaming Light, Shine on Me; Be My Friend!

You will learn about this fourth Reiki Symbol, Dai Koo Myo, during your Reiki Mastership Course. The Symbol is in many ways similar to the Power Symbol but works at a higher spiritual level. There are some more Reiki symbols added to the Reiki Mastership Course. The Tibetan Master Symbol was added much later by Mrs. Takata.

Nowadays, many Reiki Masters are coming up with their own schools of Reiki, adding more and more symbols to their system(s) of Reiki. There is nothing wrong with those but I feel all other Reiki symbols should always be used in conjunction with Dr

Usui's principal Reiki Symbols. From a personal experience, I can say that the root, the origin, is the most important. All else depends on the source sometimes the variety and the big amount of symbols added to Reiki practice may become quite confusing for the student. Dr Usui gifted us with 4 wonderful symbols, which some feel is not enough but the fact is that Dr Usui's Reiki Healing system is a complete technique with no shortcomings whatsoever. Use these symbols correctly. Love them. Trust them. And remember, we need more quality than quantity.

Chapter 15: Number Of Reiki

1. Reiki Level One: The very first Degree
Level one is a practitioner 's initiation into Reiki and it is ready to accept anyone. The emphasis throughout Level one is on opening the power channels on an actual fitness level, making it possible for the professional to hook up to the common life force energy, that passes out of the cosmos with the crown of the top and done with the center as well as hands.

Most Reiki Masters emphasize self Reiki as the aim of the Level one designation, encouraging pupils to concentrate on doing Reiki on themselves, therefore working through the own obstacles of theirs. The Reiki Level one attunement was initially provided in 4 distinct attunements. There are several Reiki Masters who however teach making use of this technique. Nevertheless, a number of Reiki Masters offer the Level one attunement in a single attunement. Lots of experience physical symptoms of electricity in the palms of theirs following the very first attunement - like tingling, heat or coolness. Generally the Level one course comes with an overview of the story of Reiki, group practice and self and hand placements.

2. Reiki Level two: Second Degree

Level two is usually identified by a focus on practicing Reiki on others, plus an expanded opening of the power channels. Furthermore students get the "Reiki symbols" and Level two attunement. The Reiki symbols let the practitioner to link deeper to the universal energy and draw on the characteristics that the symbols stand for. This includes the capability to offer distance Reiki, or driving healing energy to people anywhere they could be.

This particular symbol likewise might be utilized to clean energy blockages across time and physical locations. Because of the intensity of the attunement procedure, some Reiki Masters suggest that a minimum of twenty one days to a complete 3 months pass between getting the Level one and Level two attunements (Level one is necessary to receive Level two).

Nevertheless, you will find numerous Reiki Masters which blend Level one and Level two into a mixture type, and might even teach these throughout one weekend. The Level two attunement is normally provided in a single attunement, with a focus on opening up the main channel more, with a focus on the Heart Chakra. Usually Level two comes with train in drawing the symbols, invoking the qualities of theirs, in addition to distance healing.

3. Reiki Level three: Third Degree & Reiki Master

In courses that are many, the Third Degree and Reiki Master are exactly the same designations. However a number of teachers individual Level three from Reiki Master, to highlight the big difference in between getting the Master attunement, from becoming taught in attuning brand new pupils or even practitioners.

The Reiki Master Level is usually deemed the teacher's degree - a specialist that has gotten the power as well as expertise to attune brand new Reiki providers. Many folks get the Master attunement, together with the corresponding symbol, still do not feel at ease or even practiced in thoroughly attuning others - thus the difference between Third Degree and Reiki Master.

Turning into a Reiki Master additionally presents a full dedication to the Reiki train, as well as some believe substantial time can pass between attaining the next Degree status and Master Level. Since the Master Level is presented in a broad range of strategies, you need to meditate where path feels best for you and invest consideration and time for picking out a Master.

The Reiki Levels provide an overall organization of the development of Reiki mastership. Since Reiki programs are trained as well as organized in a number of strategies, it is essential to investigate and find both the structure as well as a teacher that's best for you.

REIKI SYMBOLS

The Reiki Symbols

Most Reiki Masters think about the Reiki symbols holy and persist in the existing Reiki tradition which they have to be kept secret. The symbols should simply be available to people who are initiated at the Reiki two levels. These days I believe that this particular strategy is no longer useful as the symbols are discussed in several books and are readily offered on the web.

Reiki symbols of no value The Reiki symbols as a result as well as the info which may be checked out about them are of very little value by themselves. In tests that are different than it's been established the symbols have little or maybe no use prior to a Reiki initiation. Pupils with absolutely no Reiki encounter (but with psychic abilities) are required to remember the symbols then use them. The outcomes differ from a management group that had Reiki two. The conclusion has been it's the Reiki initiation as a result that provides the Reiki symbols the power of theirs.

Reiki Symbols as keys The Reiki symbols are as keys which doors that are open to a greater brain. You are able to likewise see them as large buttons, whenever you press the button you instantly get an outcome. In the opinion of mine among the features of the Reiki symbols would be to immediately override the user 's precognition that a few things can't be completed (i.e. distance healing). The symbols trigger a belief or maybe purpose included in the symbols which allow the person to obtain the effects intended. The various symbols too easily join the person to the common life force.

Whenever a Reiki Master does an attunement plus displays the Reiki symbols to a pupil, the kind of sign is amazed to the pupil's head and merges with the metaphysical energies it represents.

Whenever a Reiki practitioner draws, thinks about or even visualizes a symbol it'll immediately link to the energies it provides.

3 Reiki symbols Today you will find numerous diverse kinds of Reiki and several have integrated the own symbols of theirs in the initiations of theirs. Within "traditional" Reiki you will find 3 Reiki symbols provided throughout the Reiki two Attunement (initiation). They are: the power symbol (Choku Rei), the Mental/Emotional symbol (Sei He Ki) and also the Distance symbol (Hon Sha Ze Sho Nen). You can find pictures and

information more on pages that are separate. Click on all the backlinks!

The Type Of The Symbols

The Reiki symbols are mostly based upon the Japanese writing process, Kanji. The symbols must be drawn or visualized as they've been taught throughout the Reiki two Attunement. As increasing numbers of people get attuned to Reiki this can suggest that there could be many variations in between the symbols taught by diverse Masters. This is not really a situation as there's not a hundred % right or maybe the way that is wrong to draw them. The Reiki symbols offered to a pupil is going to work the way they appear to be while they integrate the connection and the intention to the metaphysical energies it represents.

The Reiki Power symbol - Choku Rei

(Choku Rei is pronounced: "Cho-Koo-Ray") The basic significance of Choku Rei is: "Place the strength of the universe here".

The energy symbol may be utilized to boost the capability of Reiki. It is able to likewise be used for security. View it as a light switch which has the intent to immediately boost the ability of yours to channel Reiki energy.

Draw or even imagine the sign before you and also you are going to have immediate access to far more healing energies. Choku Rei additionally gives the other symbols for more power when they're used collectively.

The sign could be worn at any moment during a cure though it's particularly useful in case it's utilized at the start of any session to encourage the Reiki energy or even when utilized in the conclusion of any session to shut the session and seal off of the Reiki energies.

The Reiki Power sign is, as I've stated before, primarily a power switch though you are able to additionally assign it even further uses. Remember it's usually the intention of yours that governs what goes on. When you would like to incorporate brand new "functions" on the Power symbol next simply possess a definite intention and statement of what it's you would like the symbol to complete and yes it is going to do it for you.

Several uses:

Boost the potential of your healing abilities; use it as a gentle switch. (Draw or even visualize Choku Rei before you and bring it in the hands of yours in case you want.)

You are able to aim the Reiki energies (like a looking glass) on a certain thing of the body. (Draw the symbol on the location being treated.)

Boost the strength of the opposite symbols. (Draw it prior to drawing the other symbols.)

One may utilize the power sign in order to close an area within the receiver and also to prevent the energies got to vanish from the body. (Draw it above the entire body with the aim of sealing the healing process.)

The energy sign could be utilized to spiritually clean an area out of negative energy, to keep it in light and allow it to be a holy place. (Draw or even imagine the symbols on each one of the wall space, floor and ceiling with the intention to energize the room.)

You are able to clear other objects and crystals from bad energies. (Draw the capability sign above and on the crystal/object with the intention of purifying it and restoring it to the original state of its. Store the item in the hands of yours and "give" it Reiki (or send it Reiki from a distance in case it's way too huge to hold).)

Protect yourself from bad energies (from individuals you treat or maybe folks you meet). (Draw or even imagine the Reiki Power sign before you with the intention of being completely protected.) You are able to read about this on the page of mine regarding the "Aurashield".

Defend yourself, your spouse, your children, the house of yours along with other issues you value. (Draw Choku Rei on the object/person you wish to defend with the intention to defend him/her/it from harm.) Since Reiki works on various different levels of presence it'll normally additionally get the defense on almost all levels of existence.

These are only a couple of uses. You are able to make use of your own personal imagination and intuition to look for different uses for the Reiki Power symbol? Choku Rei. There aren't any limits to what you are able to do. The energy is actually in the mind of yours, allow your clear intention manual the performance of the symbols.

The Mental/Emotional symbol? Sei He Ki
 (Sei He Ki pronounced as: "Say-Hay-Key")
Sei He Ki has an overall meaning of: "God as well as male become one".

The Mental/Emotional symbol brings together the body" and the "brain. It can help individuals to bring to the counter and launch the mental/emotional causes of their problems.

Lots of people (even doctors) are beginning to understand that a lot of the ailments of ours are derived from emotional and mental unbalances which we most likely aren't actually conscious of. The symbol functions focusing as well as harmonize the subconscious mind with the actual physical side.

This symbol could be utilized to help with mental and emotional healing. It balances the right and left side of the mind and gives harmony and peace. It's additionally extremely effective in relationship problems. The Sei He Ki symbol could additionally be worn on several issues like nervousness, anger, depression, fear, despair etc.

Several uses:

The sign may be utilized to help you cure misuse of drugs, smoking etc, alcohol.

Sei He Ki could be utilized to lose weight.

The sign may be utilized to locate things that you've misplaced. (Draw the sign before you and also you can ask for assistance in locating XXXX. Let go of attempting to locate the object. The solution will quickly pop up.)

Sei He Ki could be utilized to improve the memory of yours when studying. and reading (Draw the symbol on every URL as you read through it with the intention of recalling the key parts.)

Include the sign when doing healing (normal or maybe distance) as this may assist the healing process. Lots of physical issues have mental/emotional roots.

The Mental/Emotional symbol, Sei He Ki, is related to Yang and Yin and also the balance between the 2 sides of the human brain.

The left portion of the sign signifies Yang and the left side of ours of the mind (logic, linear thinking etc. and structure) The proper side of the symbol symbolizes Yin and the right side of ours of the brain. (fantasy, thoughts, intuition etc.) When you're dealing with someone else and also draw the symbol on the left side of the sign, i.e. the Yang component of the sign winds up on the receiver's best side of the mind and also the Yin component on the left side therefore helping balance the 2 sides.

The Reiki Distance Healing symbol

Hon Sha Ze Sho Nen

(Hon Sha Ze Sho Nen is pronounced as: "Hon-Sha-Zee-Show-Nen")

The sign has an overall significance of: "No past, absolutely no present, without future" or maybe it is able to keep the significance of "The Buddha in my relationships the Buddha in you".

The Distance symbol can easily, as the name of its implies, be utilized to send energies with a distance. Time as well as distance is not a problem when working with this Reiki symbol. A lot of professionals regard Hon Sha Ze Sho Nen as probably the most helpful as well as an effective symbol. The utilization of the sign provides permission to access the "Akashic Records", the life records of every soul and will thus be utilized in karmic healing. Other experiences and trauma through this life, parallel or previous lives that impact and mirror peoples' habits could be brought to light and launched.

In performing distance healing be open! Don't focus the efforts of yours on healing a certain problem such as a headache. Send the Reiki energies with no limitation as they are going to go where they're best needed. When performing distance healing the energies are going to work on the receiver's subtle body, the Aura and the Chakras, without so much on the actual physical level (i.e. it is able to take the time prior to the energies seep down with the entire body and also eases for example pain).

The individual you're sending Reiki to is apt to believe it happening. In case he/she has an open mind he/she can generally tell what you've performed so when you've accomplished it.

Distance healing doesn't take almost so long as a proactive treatment. You really just require a couple of mins to post distance healing. You are able to actually create a Reiki distance healing to immediately repeat driving energies to an individual. In case you would like to accomplish this I suggest you place a time limit on the repeat (as it normally may proceed forever) and additionally to restore as well as empower the distance healing each alternate day. Remember it's the intention of yours that guides what goes on!

Several uses:

Send Reiki healing to individuals a long way away.

"Beam" Reiki to individuals across the space.

Send Reiki energies to the long term to assist with a certain job or even be there as a support.

Send Reiki on the past to raise up, to recognize as well as release trauma.

Chapter 16: The Power Of Healing

Now that we are coming to the end of this book, it is important that we close out by looking at the actual benefits that Reiki can bring us. We have talked a lot about the use and purpose, even mentioning in broad terms that it can help us to heal. But what exactly does that mean, and what are the tangible effects that people notice?

Instead of generalizing and simply saying "it heals our energy," we will break down the physical, mental, emotional, and spiritual side of Reiki and list out what it can help you to achieve. From there, we will look at how you can apply it to your own, everyday life, in order to find balance and fulfillment in each moment.

Who Can Reiki Be Used On?

Reiki can be used on anyone and everyone, with a few notable exceptions. We've talked about self-healing, and we've talked about working with clients, but what about babies or animals?

● **Pregnant Women** – During pregnancy, we undergo a multitude of changes, both physically and emotionally. Reiki is completely safe to practice on pregnant women, and will not have any negative effect on the growing baby inside of her. In fact, Reiki can actually make pregnancy much more enjoyable and can help alleviate many of the negative symptoms that pregnant women experience. For example:

● It can reduce or prevent morning sickness

● It can reduce inflammation and swelling in places like the ankles

● It can minimize stiffness, aches, and pains

● It can make women feel more awake and less tired

● It helps to strengthen the bond between mother and child

- It can help reduce the risk of postpartum depression
- It helps to protect and nurture the unborn baby
- **Babies –** Once the baby is born, Reiki can be used on infants in order to help them with their development, connection to the new world, and treat any post-birth conditions. Some of the ways it can treat babies is by:
- Help to balance the baby's energy
- Reduce the stress caused by the birthing process
- Promote healthy sleeping habits
- Charging the breast milk or formula with healing energy
- Create a strong bond between baby and parents
- Treat conditions such as colic or cradle cap
- **Children –** As the baby grows into a child, they can still benefit from Reiki treatments in their life. From toddlers to teenagers, Reiki can help with the stress of

growing up and to instill confidence and self-worth within a child. Just like with adults, it can help them with any illness or ailment, as well as any emotional turmoil they experience during times like puberty or entering school.

● **Animals –** We often forget that animals undergo many of the same things we do, and they can be overcome by physical or even emotional ailments. Animals are surprisingly sensitive to Reiki, and so it is worthwhile to practice on your pets so that they, too, can reap all of the healing benefits.

● **Plants and Vegetation –** If you are an avid gardener, Reiki can actually help you to grow the garden of your dreams. You should notice that after doing Reiki on plants that they flourish and grow strong, bearing beautiful flowers or ripe fruit.

Now, there are a small group of individuals who should not seek out Reiki treatment, due to the fact that it can have an adverse reaction. These include:

- Individuals who have a pacemaker, as it can interfere with how it works
- People who are contagious should not have Reiki done in person
- If someone is intoxicated, you should never perform a session on them
- Those with a fever should avoid Reiki as it can increase the body temperature
- If someone is driving or operating heavy machinery, they should not undergo Reiki at that moment
- People who have broken a bone which has not yet been set should not receive Reiki
- Distance healing for those who are actively in surgery should be avoided as it can interfere with the anesthesia

Other than that, which has been listed, everyone else is free to receive Reiki as they wish, and it will do no harm whatsoever.

Physical Healing

When we conduct a Reiki treatment session, there are genuine physical benefits that arise from this. Reiki doesn't need to only be discussed in broad terms, and we can actually pinpoint the exact ways in which healing can occur. But what exactly can we expect to accomplish physically? Here is a list of possible physical disorders that can be treated during a Reiki session:

- Specific pain: such as that which occurs in the back, neck, shoulders, or legs
- General pain: such as an overall ache or tightness throughout all of the muscles
- Headaches and migraines
- Thyroid and hormonal imbalances
- Chronic fatigue and insomnia
- Skin conditions such as eczema or psoriasis
- Oral conditions such as gingivitis or TMJ
- Cancer in various stages
- Autoimmune disorders
- Post-surgery recovery
- Digestive issues and bowel problems such as IBS
- Calms nausea

- Removes tension from the body
- Reduce and prevent heart disease and stroke
- Help with infertility issues
- Assists those suffering from neurodegenerative disorders
- Works on Crohn's disease
- Vision and sight problems
- Hearing loss
- Hair loss and thinning
- Can reduce inflammation associated with arthritis
- Increase mobility and range of motion
- Heals infections
- Used for those with metabolic syndrome
- Reduces symptoms of diabetes
- And much more…

Reiki isn't a magic cure, and if you are suffering from acute symptoms, you should always consult your medical practitioner to discuss your options. But, when used in conjunction with conventional medicine, it can speed up healing, promote overall wellness, and help to stop the progression of many diseases. There is no harm to adding Reiki into your treatment plan, so see if it can help you with both acute and long term illnesses.

Mental Healing

Just like with the list of ways that Reiki can help physically, there are also a number of different mental conditions in which Reiki can be beneficial. From specific disorders to generalized concerns, there is a lot that can be done via a session. Before you use Reiki for mental healing, however, it is recommended that you consult a health care practitioner that is trained in this area. Reiki cannot diagnose an illness and instead can only help to treat it. If you are unsure if you are suffering from a diagnosable mental illness, you should get that looked at prior to Reiki treatment. Some of the conditions that can be helped by Reiki include:

- Generalized Anxiety Disorder
- Social Anxiety

- Major Depressive Disorder caused by imbalances
- Bipolar Disorder
- Seasonal Affective Disorder
- Obsessive Compulsive Disorder
- Borderline Personality Disorder
- Schizophrenia
- Panic Disorder
- Other major mood disorders
- Psychotic disorders with hallucinations and delusions
- Impulse Control Disorders such as pyromania and kleptomania
- Post-Traumatic Stress Disorder
- Fears and phobias
- Paranoia
- Overcoming addiction or alcoholism
- Drug and alcohol withdrawal
- Brain damage
- Epilepsy
- Chronic fatigue
- Recovery from anesthesia
- Headaches and migraines
- Promotes calmness and relaxation

- Added mental clarity
- Suicide prevention
- Overcoming trauma
- Eating disorders such as anorexia and bulimia
- ADD and ADHD
- Burnout in mental health professionals
- And much more…

There is some overlap between physical disorders and mental disorders, and that is due to the fact that all processes within the body are interconnected. Many mental health concerns also present with physical symptoms, just as physical ailments can create mental health problems. As we will see in the next section, there is even more overlap when discussing emotional healing, as our emotions and our mental health and the most closely linked together. The reason they are in different categories; however, is because no all emotional troubles are mental health disorders. A person can feel sad without meeting the criteria for depression, just as they can be worried about an upcoming event without having true anxiety. These are very important distinctions because treating emotional issues will be a different process than treating someone who is diagnosed with a mental health disorder.

Emotional Healing

As we said, emotional healing can be done on anything that plays on our emotions, and this doesn't always mean that someone is suffering from a diagnosed mental health condition. In order to be diagnosed with a disorder, individuals need to meet a variety of criteria for that to be done. But we all experience emotional turmoil in our lives, and Reiki can help us overcome those feelings and to process them. Some of the emotional aspects that Reiki works on include:

- Depression triggered by a specific event such as the death of a loved one
- Grief
- General sadness

- Anger issues
- Daily stresses
- Anxiety about an upcoming event
- Worrying about the future
- General uneasiness
- Annoyance towards friends, family, and children
- Guilt stemming from past actions
- Low self-esteem and self-worth
- Disappointment in yourself and others
- Shame or embarrassment in yourself
- Loneliness
- Feeling stuck in life
- Lack of motivation and drive
- Feeling discouraged
- Apathy and feeling nothing at all
- Frustration with others or with life in general
- Contempt or jealousy
- Overinflated sense of ego
- Aggressive and overbearing emotions
- Uncontrollable jealousy
- Nervousness that affects our ability to do things

- Feeling on edge all of the time
- Unable to create a sense of peace or calmness
- Restlessness that affects sleep
- Past abandonment issues
- Overcoming an accident or injury
- Unresolved issues relating to childhood
- Feelings after a relationship ends
- Being humiliated in public
- Emotions stemming from bullying
- And much more…

As you can see, these differ from what was listed under mental healing as they are conditions and moments that most of us experience from time to time. Many of us will not be diagnosed with mental illness, but most of us will have a relationship end, experience bullying, or have to deal with the death of a loved one. These occurrences create a huge emotional impact on us and can be difficult to deal with on our own. That is why Reiki for emotional healing can be so powerful, as it brings these emotions to the surface and allows us to face them head on and with the help of a trained Reiki practitioner.

Spiritual Healing

This last aspect of Reiki healing is the one that is the most commonly referred to, and yet the one that people disagree with the most. Those who come into the path of Reiki are all different people with varying backgrounds and belief systems. Not everyone will believe in a God, deities, or even a higher being, so it can be tough to explain the spiritual benefits to someone who doesn't believe in spirituality. While most people you encounter within Reiki will have some faith or spirituality, this isn't true for all, and that is important to remember. Even if someone doesn't believe, however, they can still reap all of the spiritual healing that is open to them. Some of the spiritual situations that Reiki can work on include:

- Past life healing
- Connecting with a divine entity
- Opening and balancing the chakras

- Realigning the chi, prana, or life energy
- Balancing of the mind and the emotions
- Promote harmony within the soul
- Awaken a person spiritually
- Give guidance and increase intuition
- Increase psychic abilities and clairvoyance
- Lift the veil between this world and the next
- Creates a deeper sense of relaxation and calms the mind
- Removes any negative energy from the body
- Used to ground and center
- Promotes spiritual growth
- Helps a person learn and acknowledge their truth
- Increases our capability to love unconditionally
- Connects us and allows us to see the universe and interconnected
- Transforms time and space
- Inspires change within us
- Affects and can help us see the future

- Keeps you on your destined spiritual life plan
- Draws positivity and opportunities towards you
- Purify your karma and support the creation of good karma
- Connect to enlightened beings
- Rejuvenate the aura
- Access past or forgotten memories
- And much more...

There are virtually endless possibilities when it comes to Reiki healing, and that is why it is worthwhile that everyone experiences a session at least once in their lifetime. Whether you end up continuing with it is up to you, but at least see what effect it can have on you as you grow and develop in this life.

Even if you never end up practicing, you can incorporate the teachings of Reiki into your everyday life, and learn how to live with more compassion, more kindness, and more love. This world can get very dark, and we have the power to be a light in that darkness, guiding ourselves and others towards a better future. Never underestimate the gifts that already exist within you, and simply need to be tapped into in order to reap the benefits. Reiki is a divine wisdom and energy that has always existed and will continue to always exist, ensuring that humans are always able to create a better path for themselves and others.

So, throw caution to the wind, open up your mind, and discover an entirely new way of thinking. One in which you are no longer controlled by external sources and negative emotions, but instead feel a newfound sense of freedom and happiness. Reiki will transform who you are and how you see the world, making your time on this earth as positive and enjoyable as possible.

Chapter 17: Spiritual Connections

The Rei or God consciousness guides the Reiki healing sessions to create any changes that need to be made in this spiritual process, depending on the receiver's needs. Life holds many opportunities and experiences, some good and some challenging. When you use Reiki as a spiritual path, you will begin to actually see your energy come to life. Thinking, seeing, and doing positive things as well as using meditation to help accomplish goals, remove anger and aggression, as well as sadness and depression, and will allow you to visualize solutions that you may have otherwise missed. This will keep your outlook in a positive frame of mind.

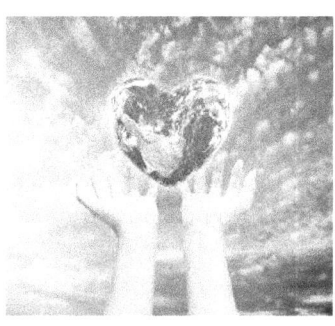

When people are faced with serious illness or disease, they will often tell you that they walk forward, not dwelling on the road they have just traveled. They simply continue to put one foot in front of the other. Negativity will destroy people, they will have defeat in their minds and hearts, and that is a powerful thing. If you believe you can't make it or do it, then you won't.

Reiki not only provides the correct information, but also the right kind of personal energy needed to take the required actions. Our lives are created from effects of all those actions we have taken and decisions we have made in this life and in past ones. Every action has an effect which comes back to us eventually. If we accept the philosophy and the fact that we are responsible for everything we do in life, then we will be centered in our power and be better able to create change in our life that is both positive and long-lasting.

Reiki should be a ritual you perform on a regular schedule, and also spontaneously if you feel the need. If you listen to your breath, your heart, mind and body, you will find the feeling of spiritual wellbeing that you are looking for. When this happens, keep in mind that everyone around you will reap the benefits as well.

People are created in all sizes and shapes, backgrounds, ethnicities, but we are all one family with spiritual souls that can be damaged but healed as well. The key to spiritual wellness is positivity, happiness, and love. Reiki will surround you and your whole entire life with a radiant glow of energy creating love and hope and, as a byproduct, a healthy body and mind as well.

This amazing spiritual path will lead you and connect you to the wisdom and power that is within you. You have always had a plan, you just somehow didn't know what it was before your spiritual connection showed you the way. By healing and releasing everything that is blocking your path, you will be truly healed and filled with everything positive and good, not to mention a magnitude of energy you cannot begin to imagine.

Your true spiritual path is always there, but sometimes, others will try intentionally or unintentionally to make you feel their pain and problems. Some people have negative issues and somehow feel better if everyone has that negativity as well. You do not have to feel their pain and cope with their problems because you have a better plan, a highly powerful spiritual plan that is always there when you need it the most. This is a wonderful part of living with Reiki's energy. Remember, don't let anyone place negativity on your beautiful path. Do what you love to do and cherish what you love. It is powerful, healing, and healthy.

Negativity Eraser – Take 5! *(5 minutes)*

When you are stressed with limited time, getting the kids off to school, job project scheduling, appointments to set, find five minutes to erase these pressures from your mind. Just for five minutes do a powerful and positive thing for yourself. Stop and "take 5!"

Find a quiet space. Even if you put headphones on to keep the outside world, out. A walk, a park bench, a corner in a coffee shop, a library, a park. Sit and just breathe. Slow, long breaths, in and out. Your mind is full... move negativity out.

In your mind, think of a pen and paper or a chalkboard.

You need to mentally write your stressors down.

With your eyes closed, take deep slow breaths in and out, in and push gently on the back of the air to push it out.

Now in your mind, you can see the chalk in your hand and visualize it moving to the board.

See all of the stress-filled "stuff" in a pile; things are moving from your mind to the top of the pile.

One after another.

Visualize them each going out of the top of your head and floating to the top of a pile. Each item is then written on the board using your hand that is holding the chalk.

You are aware of this, but you are unaware of your hand moving.

You see an eraser that is beginning to remove each stressful item one by one.

Watch them disappear. And with each one that is erased, feel positive energy entering your body.

The stress is gone; school stress is gone; job stress is gone, one right after another, gone!

Still, with rhythmic calming breathing, visualize a clean board.

It doesn't even have a trace of dust on it.

Your mind feels light but strong. The burdens have disappeared.

All you can feel is your calming breath.

Things are just "things." Your mind and body will help you to put "things" in order. "You" are what is most important in the world! You are at a serious health risk if you don't take care of yourself.

Do this simple meditation exercise every day. Only 5 minutes and you will be amazed at the positive outcome that will "erase" the negativity. Soon you will not have anything to erase!

The gift of Reiki is a spiritual one that helps to transform you for the better. When you decide you want to become a Reiki practitioner, you will be connected directly to a powerful, divine energy healing source, and that will be able to flow healing energy through your hands for the rest of your life. This practice is applied to thousands of people all over the globe. Reiki is a completely safe, unbelievably easy and powerful part of giving and receiving healing energy through spiritual interconnectedness.

By using First Degree Reiki, a connection is created for healing energy that will start the flow of powerful energy healing to ourselves and others. This healing process can't be misused or abused as it is similar to a pure filter of the divine healing energy that flows all through the attuned person's hands and onto the patient. Reiki is really an extraordinary gift of the divine that can assist people that are on a spiritual journey in order to bring healing balance to all parts of our spiritual, emotional, mental, and physical bodies.

The more that spiritual and energy healing are applied, the clearer the channels will be and the better you will become at manipulating the energy. Also, we are more balanced and healed when we are channeling ourselves. An awakening self-healing journey will make us better and stronger healers. The path of balance, happiness, and healing has to be cultivated with wisdom and love, and will therefore, align us with the principles from the divine that will allow us to release the pain and fear we have been holding onto, possibly for years. Energy healing also gives us more confidence and self-assurance and awareness of the positive changes around us and in our lives as we become healthier and happier.

For many people, First Degree Reiki is the beginning of a new start in life. It also may be the start of a new spiritual journey of discovery and challenging insight. These journeys have taught others that things will happen to us, but the way that we view others and the life surrounding us are reflections of ourselves. The world is showing us these reflections so we can see ourselves and our pain, fear, wisdom, and love. It makes us see who we are and gives us a knowledge of life that is a part of ourselves, our souls, and our awareness of who we are. Our ability to think clearly brings thoughts of deep healing to us, so we are able to have and live in greater harmony with the universe.

For the people that seek Reiki to pursue its healing powers, it is an emotionally spiritual part of their lives. It is believing that wisdom and spiritual truth is in all the major parts of the universe we live in and also believing that they will ultimately lead to paths that will take you to the same place. For many, Reiki can heighten their spiritual feelings of peace without any negativity because it is a divine thread which connects us and that does not have any attached doctrine. People who feel they are spiritual but not really religious can be connected by the Reiki attunement as a feeling of the divine creation.

A human's soul is amazing and complex in a way that connects the body with the mind. We need to understand that we are rewarded by teachings and healing, and in the end, they free us from pain and fear in order to achieve spiritual healing and lasting growth. This knowledge is very useful to those who want to advance in any way possible. Great faith and an incredibly deep-rooted belief show us that when a person wants or needs to change to a positive emotional state, then the soul will figure out a way to get there.

Conclusion

Thank you for making it through to the end of this book and let's hope it was informative and able to provide you with all of the tools you need to achieve your goals, whatever they may be.

Everything begins with our own health. Whether it is in our personal or career lives, our well-being adds to our everyday outlook and our emotional and physical health. Reiki will add energy to create a more peaceful life, resulting in a happier, more productive life. The more you use the powerful force of Reiki, the more you will feel balanced!

The biggest benefit of Reiki healing treatment is that this treatment increases your energy power to help heal others and yourself quickly. By promoting relaxation, creating a peaceful feeling, and reducing your stress, you will begin to shift yourself forward toward your unique spiritual, mental, and physical balance and experience your own body's healing mechanisms beginning to work more effectively.

Reiki is a non-invasive way to bring positive energy forces that will create mind and body wellness. It is an amazing feeling when this energy surrounds you and flows through your body and mind while you concentrate on wellness. It is a powerful tool that will change and improve your life while inspiring you to change and focus on a healthy body and mind.

Reiki's powerful and mystic force flows in and out of your physical body using crossings known as "chakras," feeding your organs and cells as they make their way through every part of your body and mind to keep you well and healthy.

When this force is interrupted or blocked, the areas that are affected can stop functioning and will be detrimental to your health, which could cause illness or even worse, a devastating disease. Reiki is a powerful way to stop this blockage and help to keep that life force energy working to keep you healthy.

www.ingramcontent.com/pod-product-compliance
Lightning Source LLC
Chambersburg PA
CBHW072008070526
44583CB00015B/1391